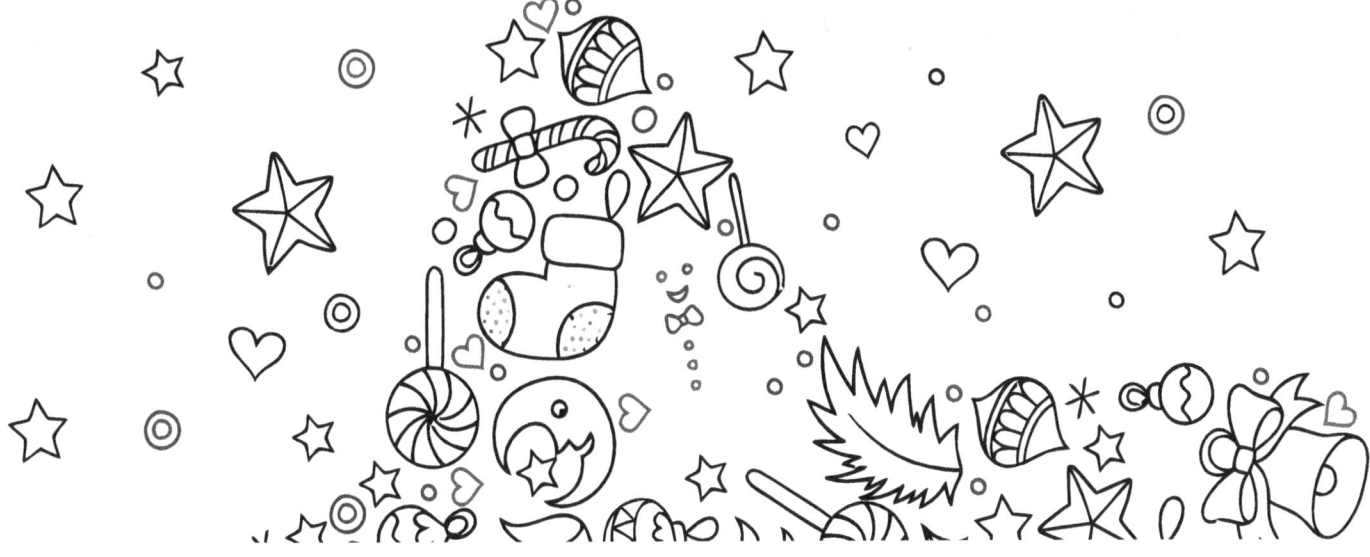

This Christmas Coloring Book
Belongs To:

_____

_____

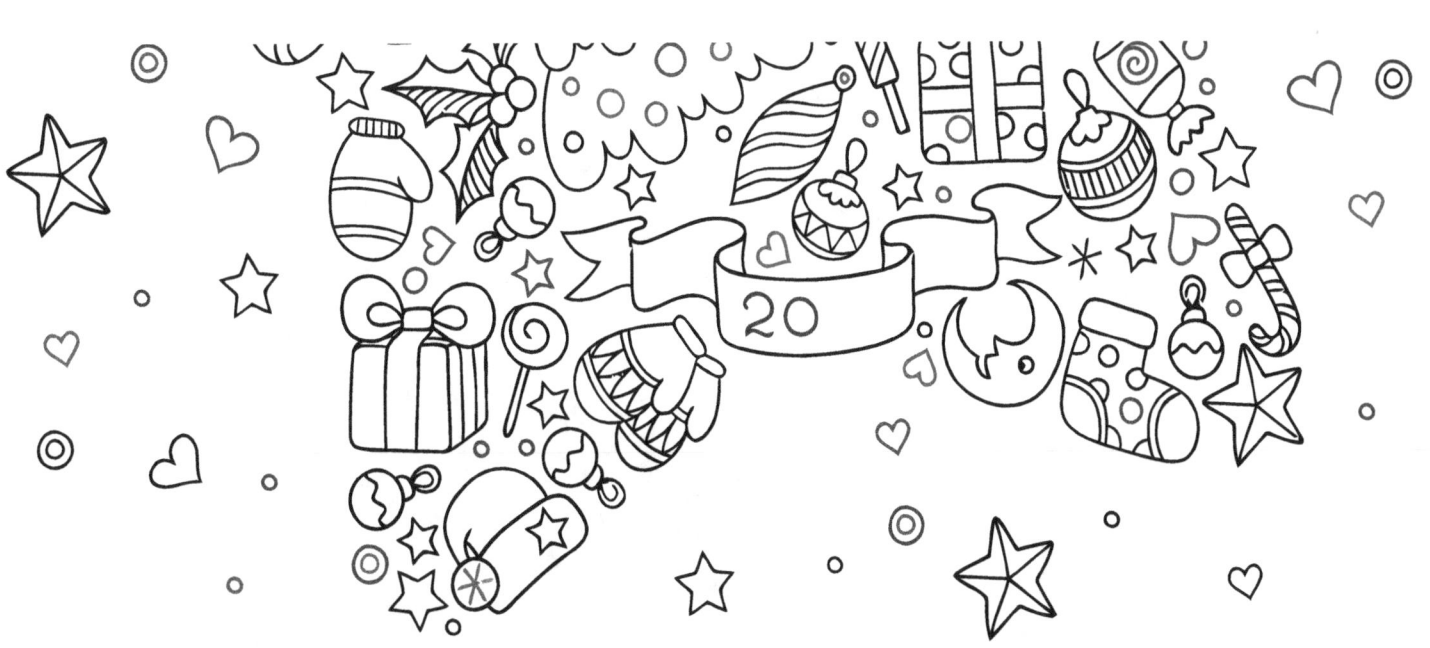

Write and Draw to Express Yourself

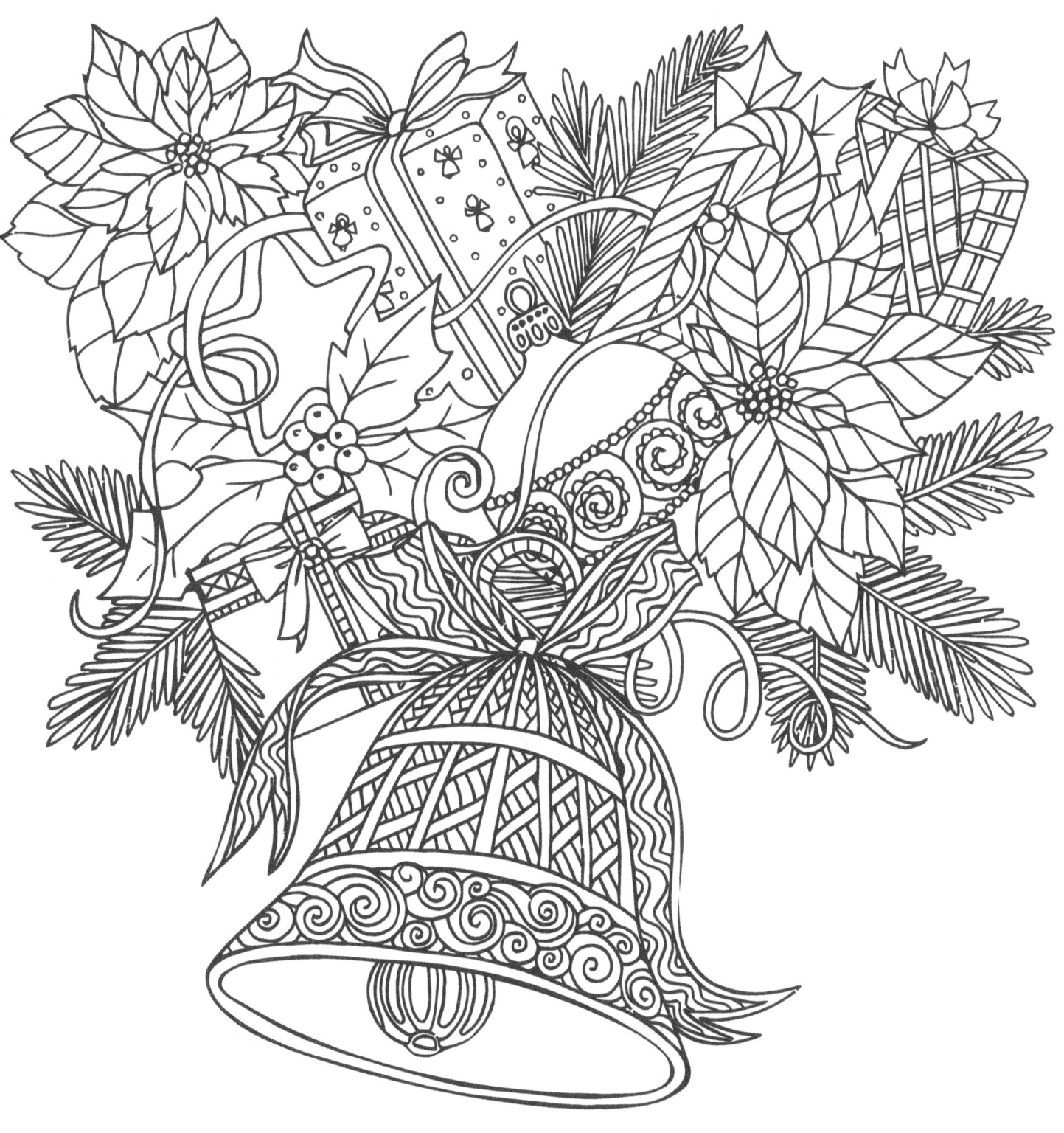

Write and Draw to Express Yourself

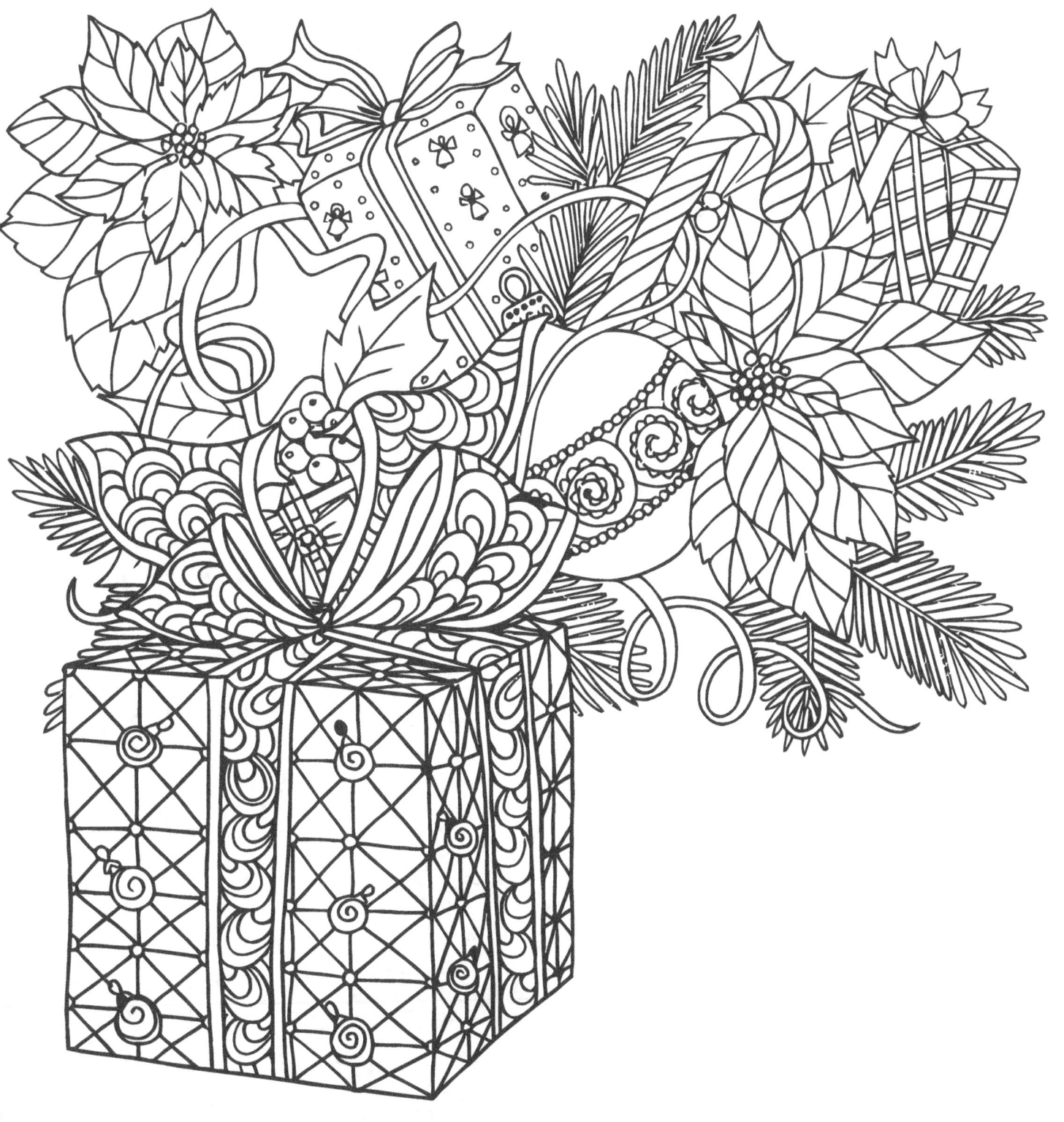

Write and Draw to Express Yourself

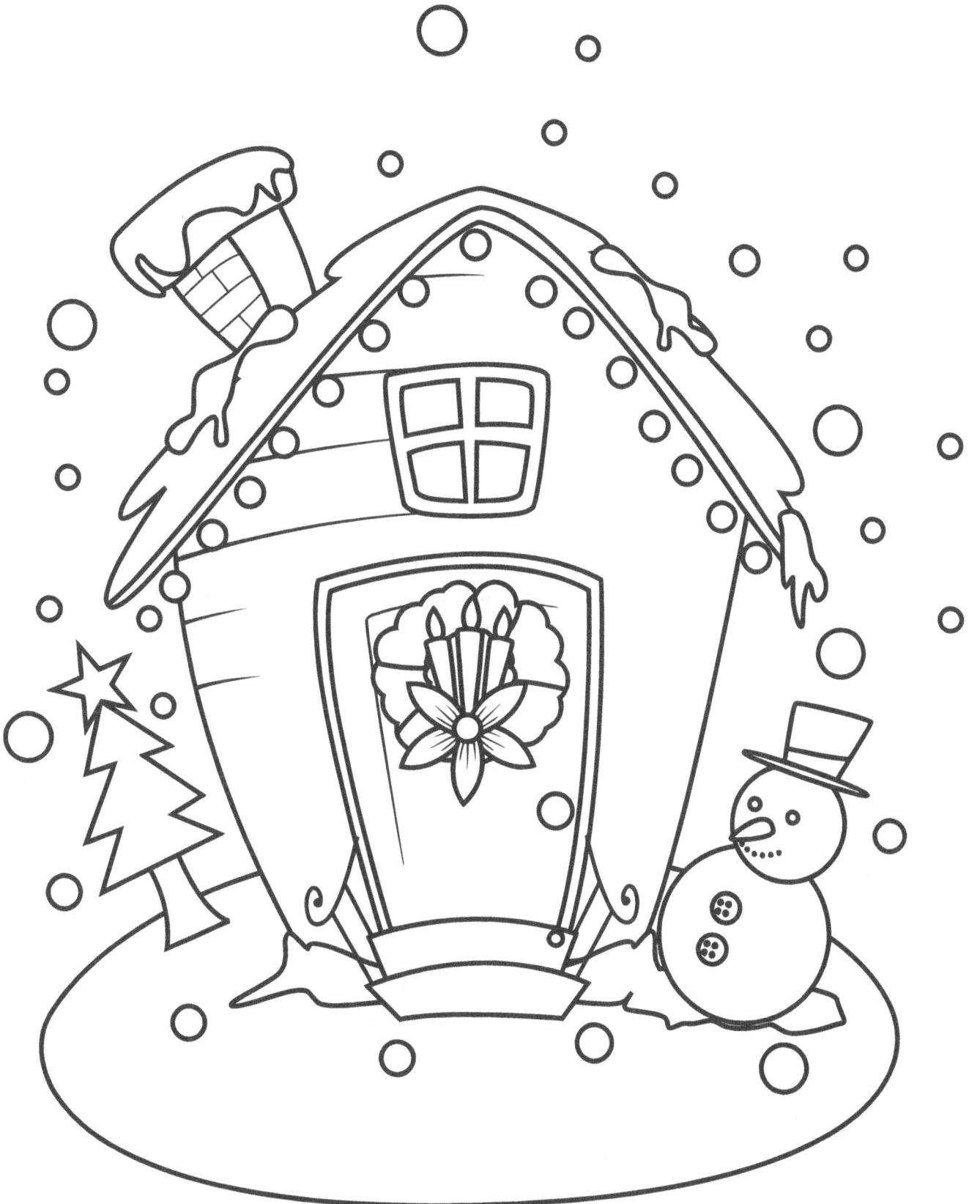

Write and Draw to Express Yourself

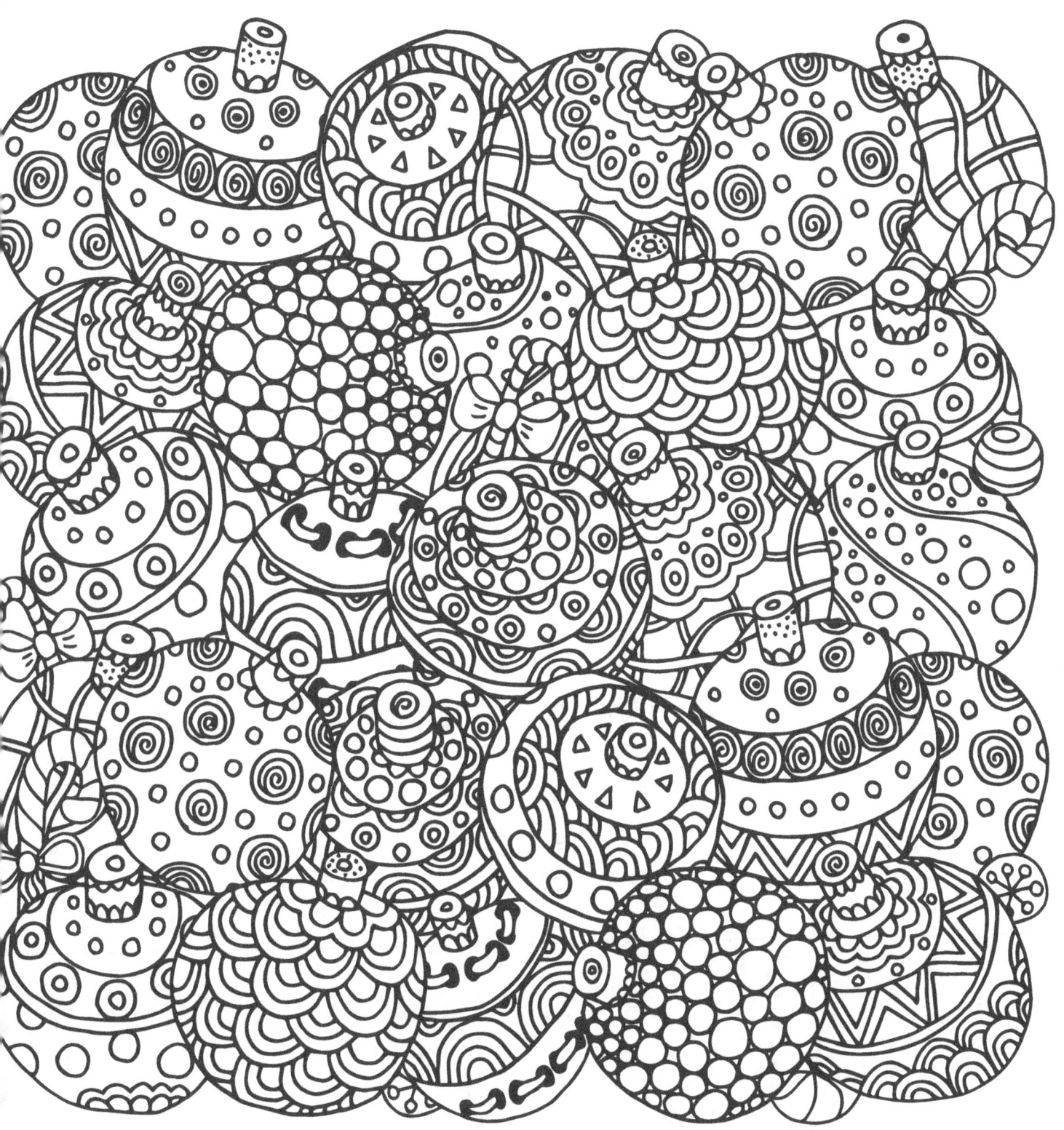

Write and Draw to Express Yourself

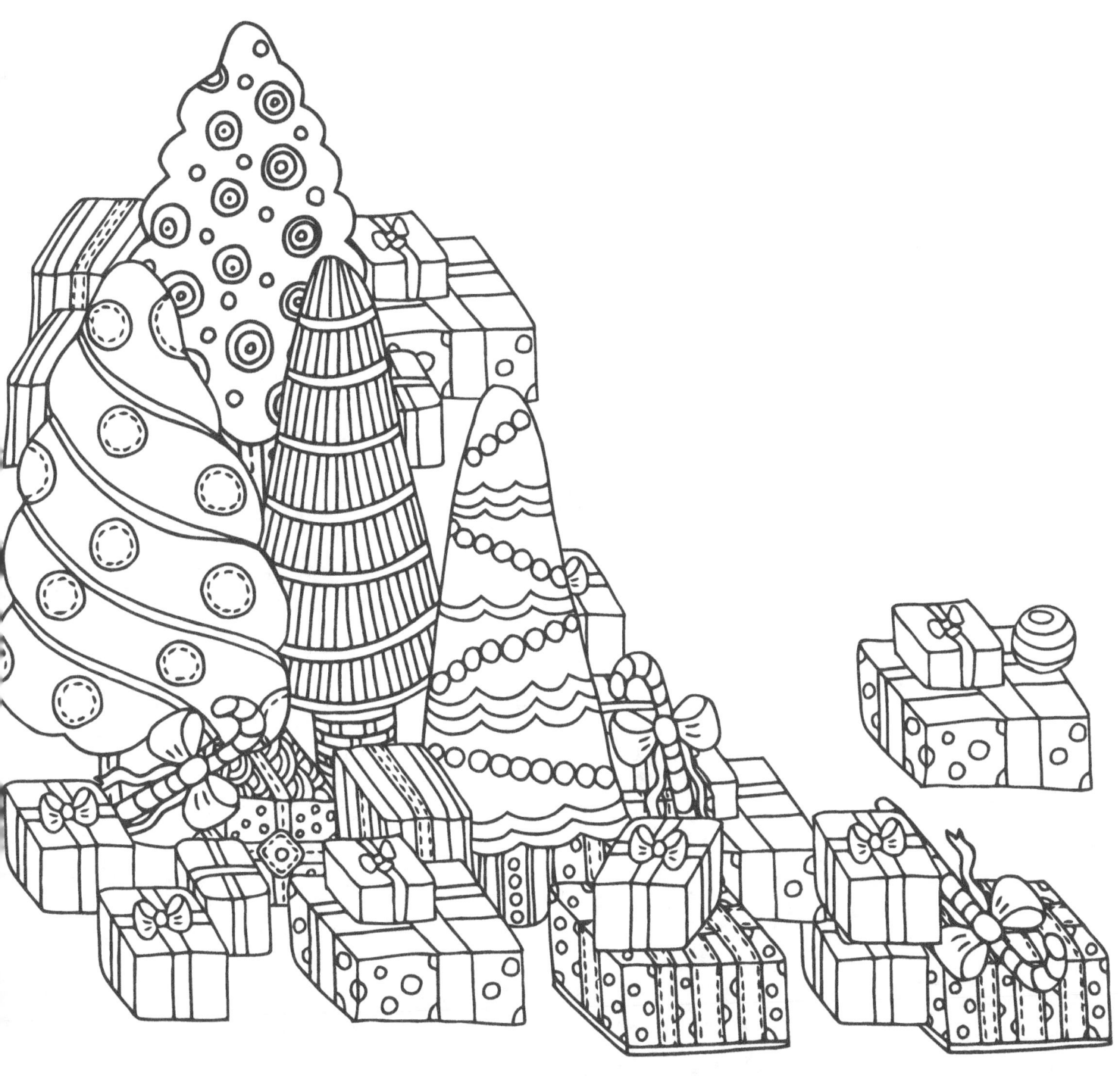

Write and Draw to Express Yourself

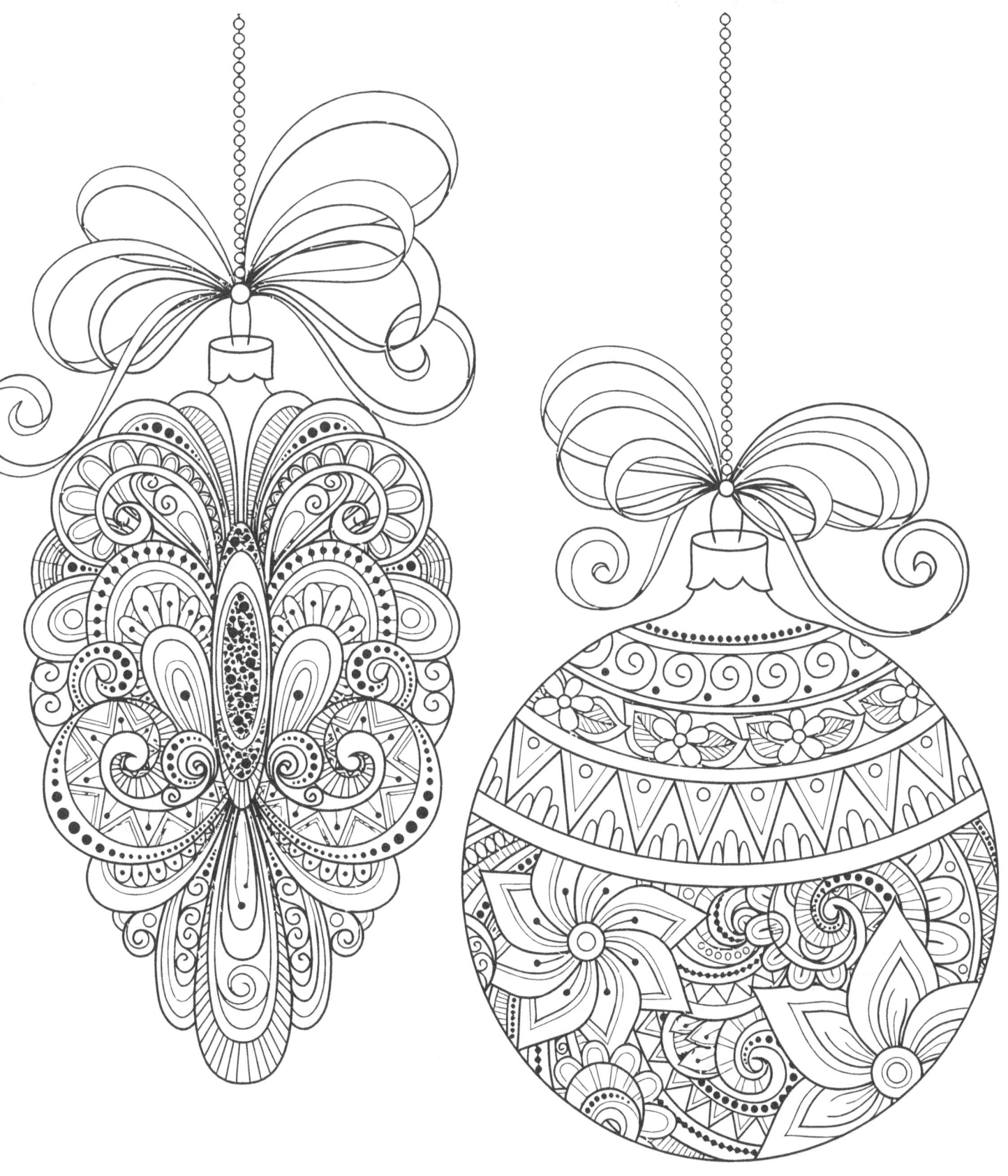

Write and Draw to Express Yourself

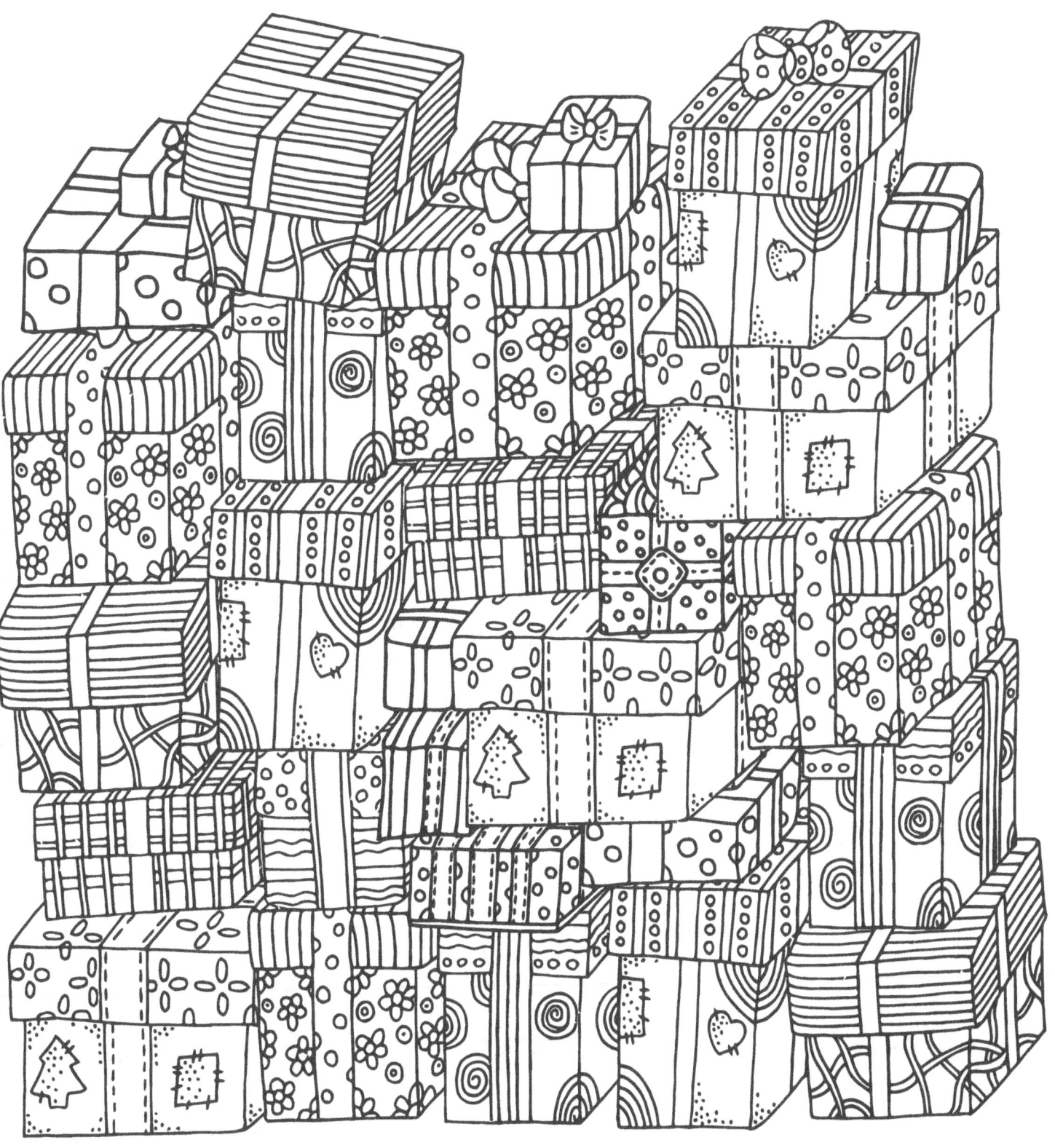

Date: ____ / ____ / ____

Write and Draw to Express Yourself

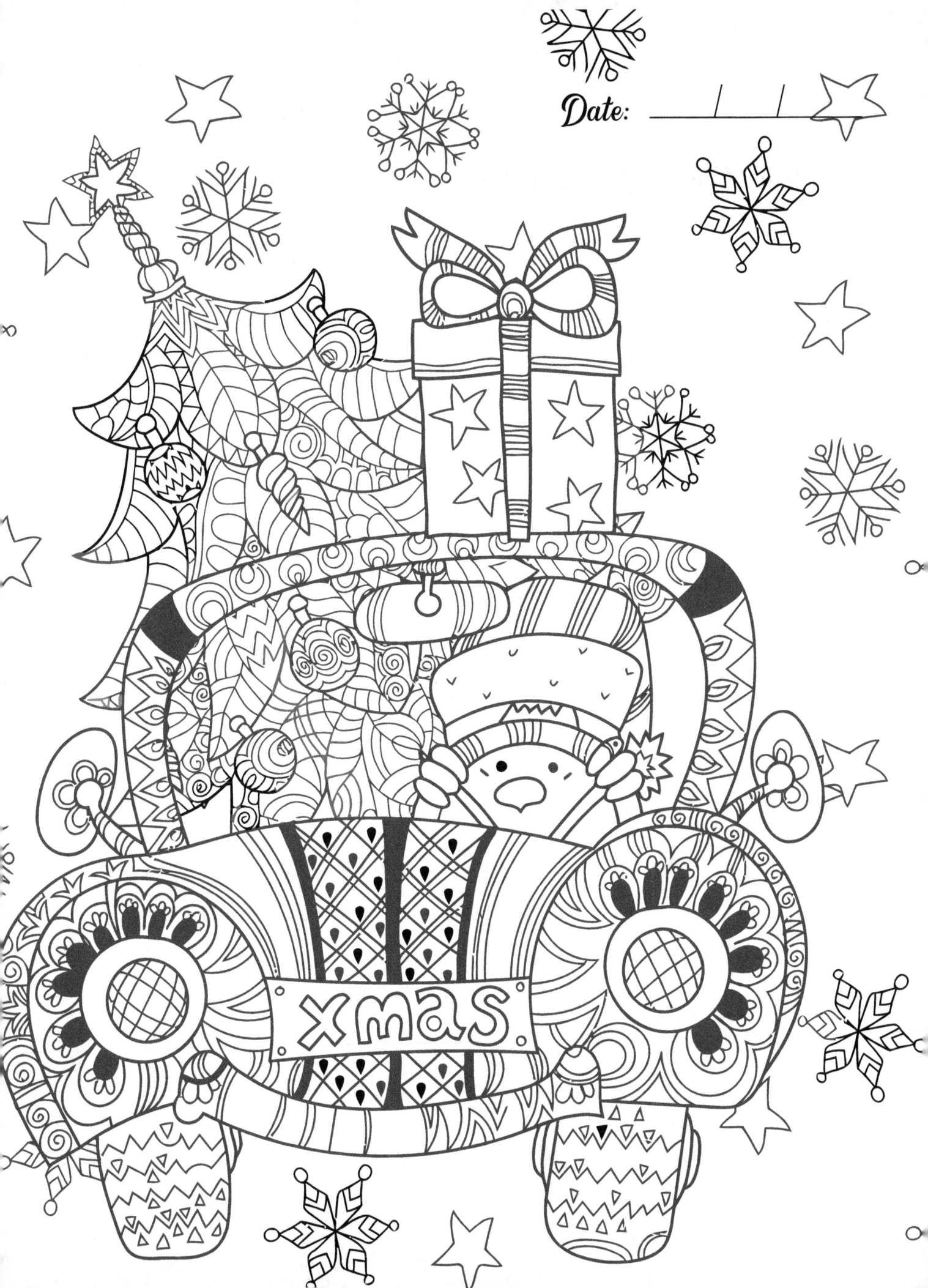

Write and Draw to Express Yourself

Date: _____

Write and Draw to Express Yourself

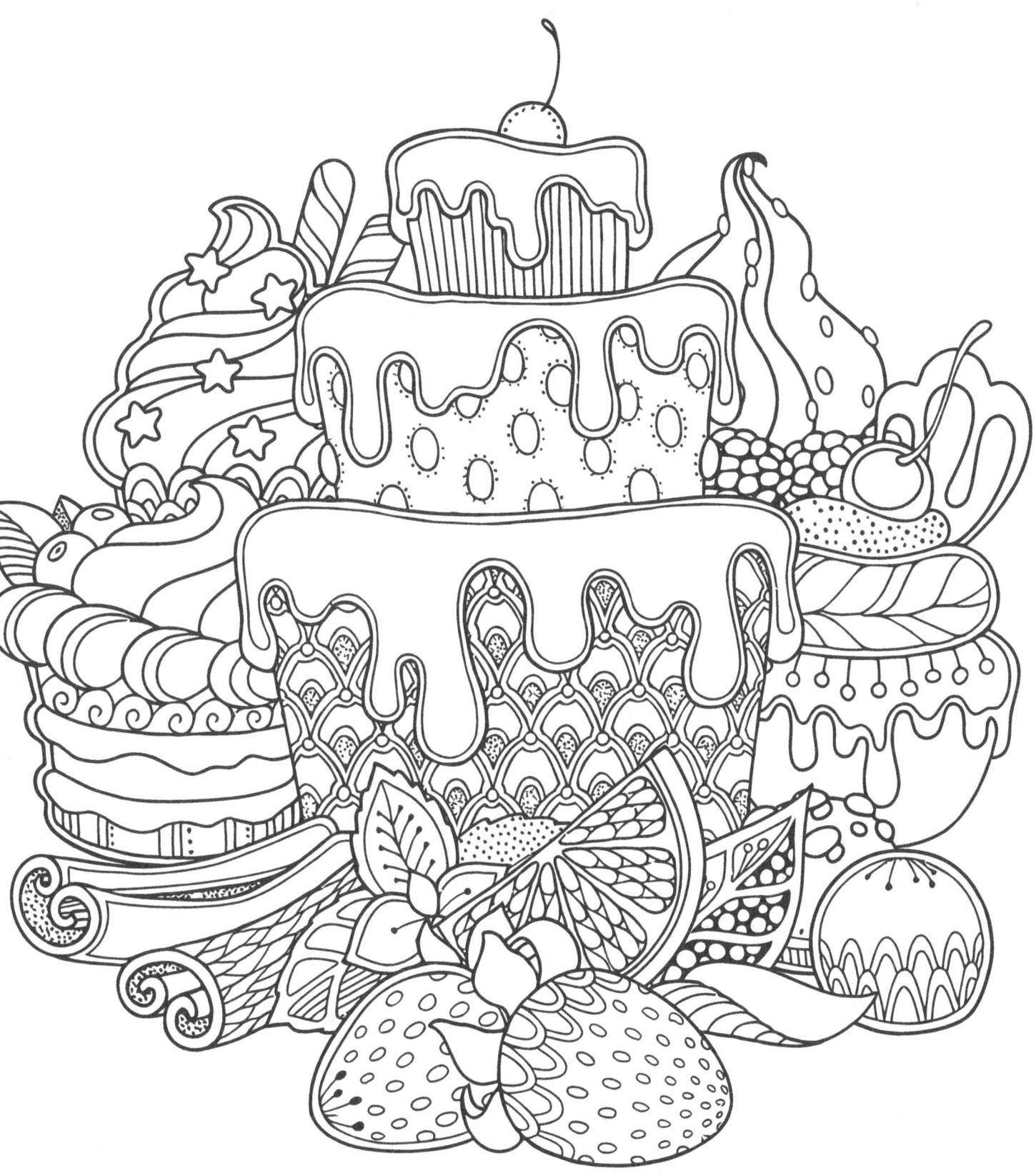

Write and Draw to Express Yourself

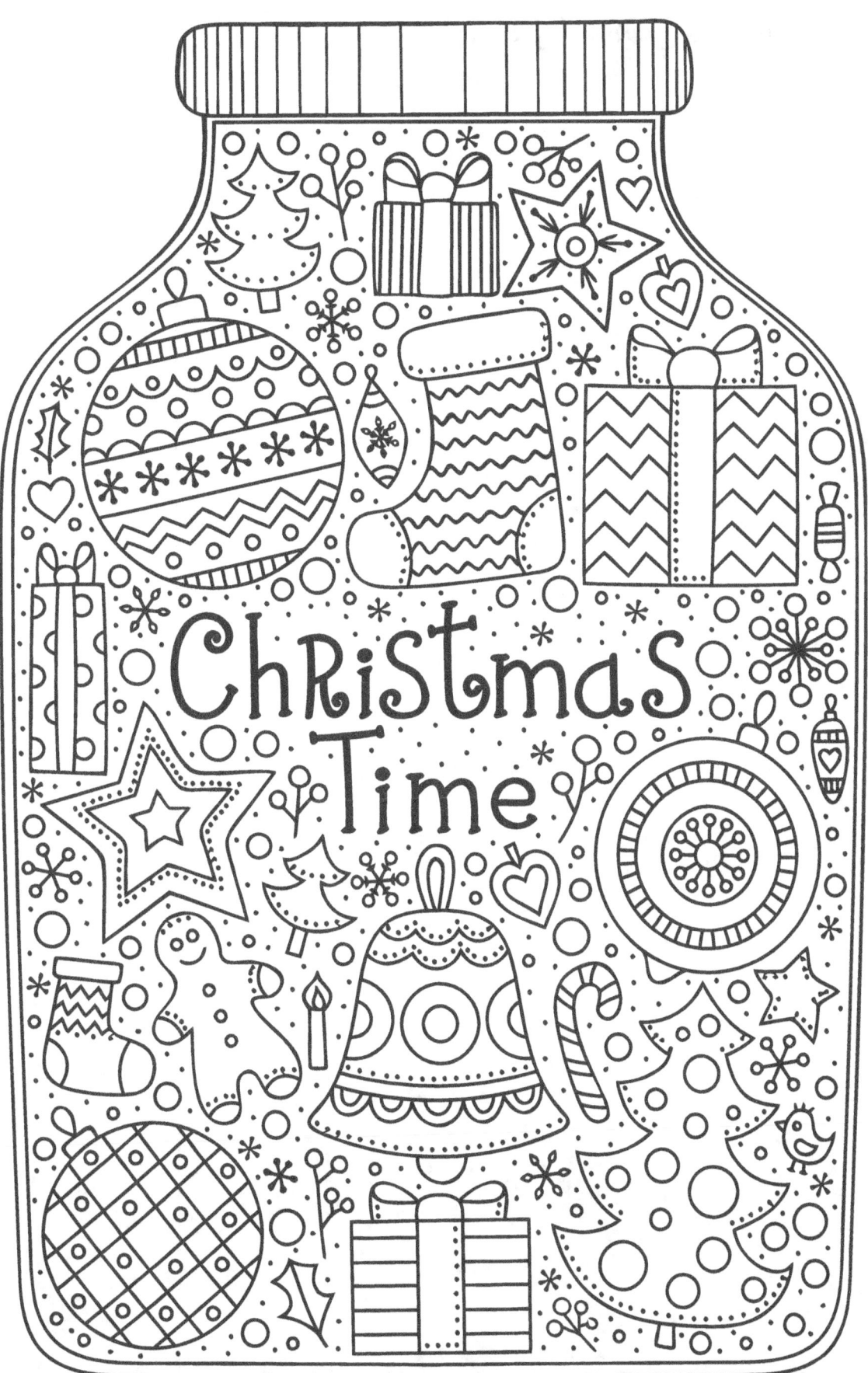

Write and Draw to Express Yourself

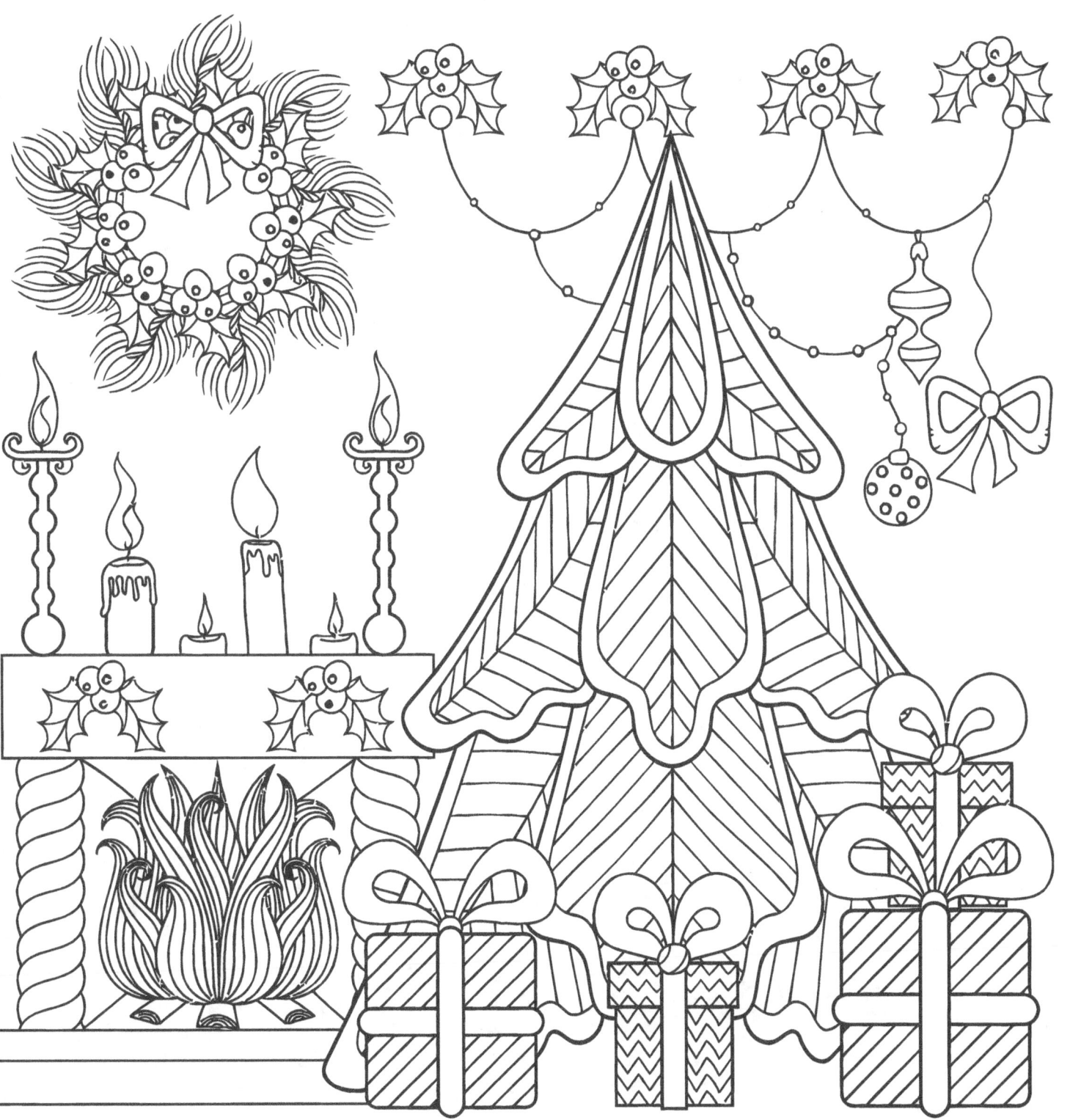

Write and Draw to Express Yourself

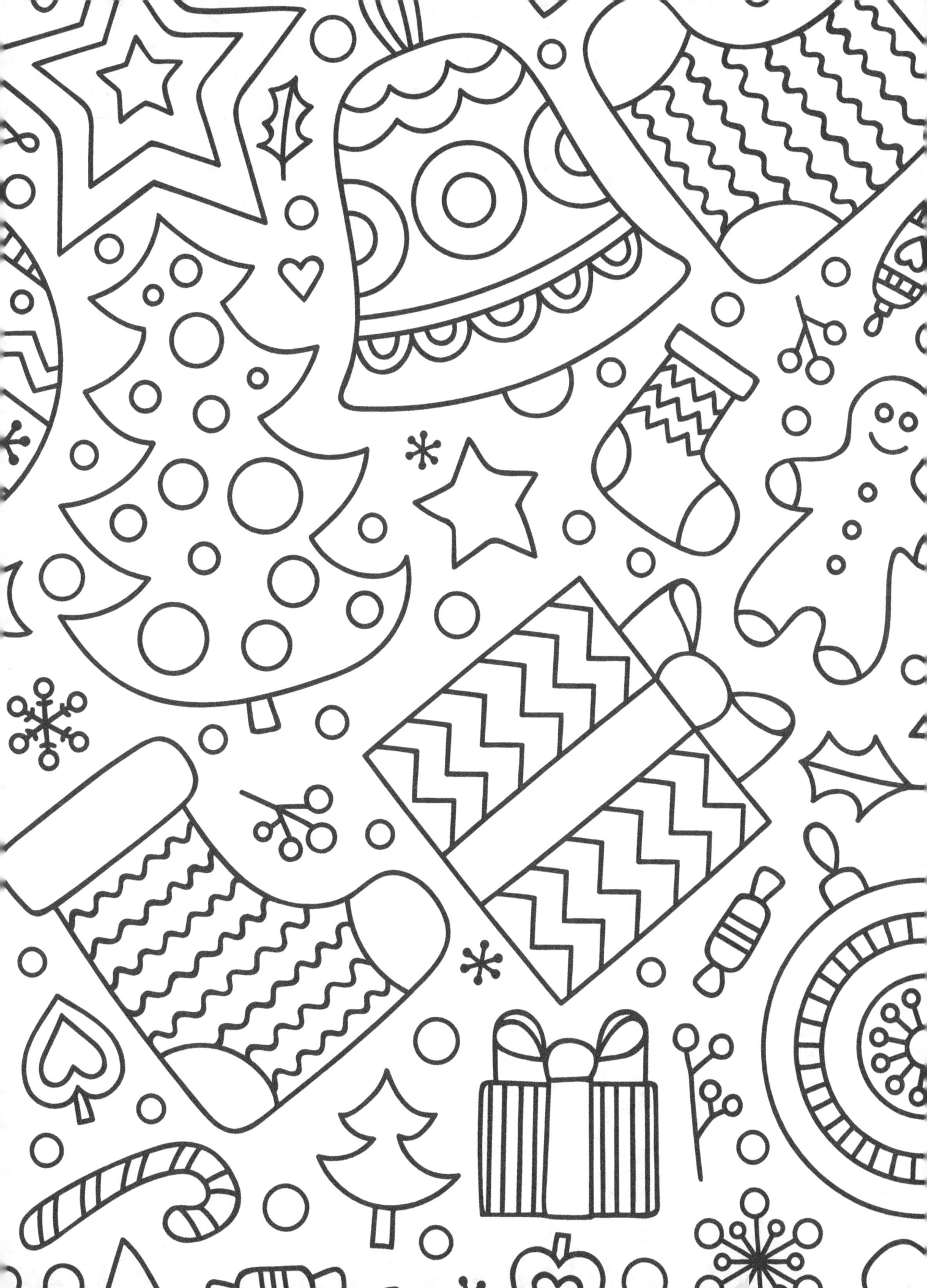

Write and Draw to Express Yourself

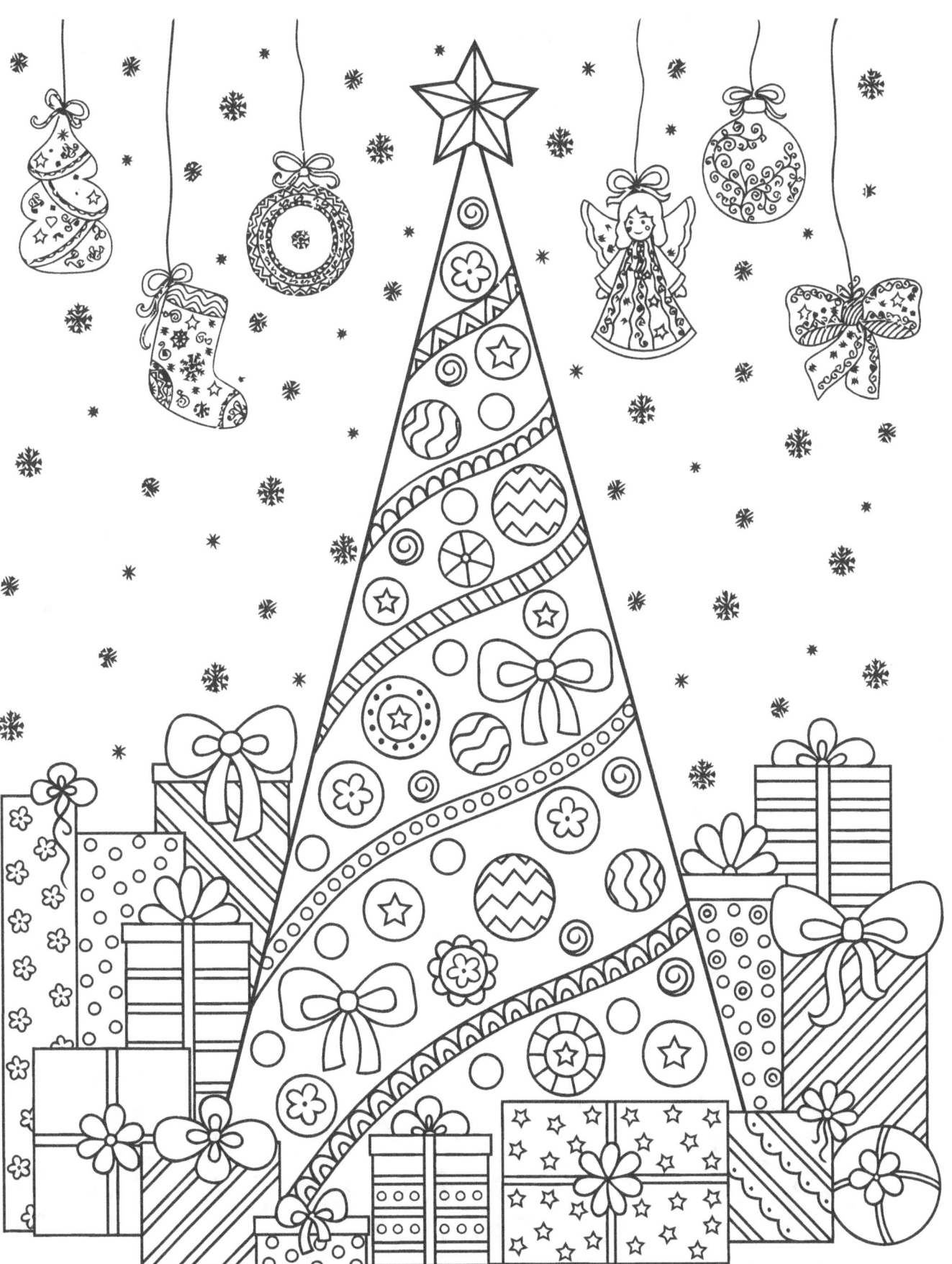

Date: ___/___/___

Write and Draw to Express Yourself

Write and Draw to Express Yourself

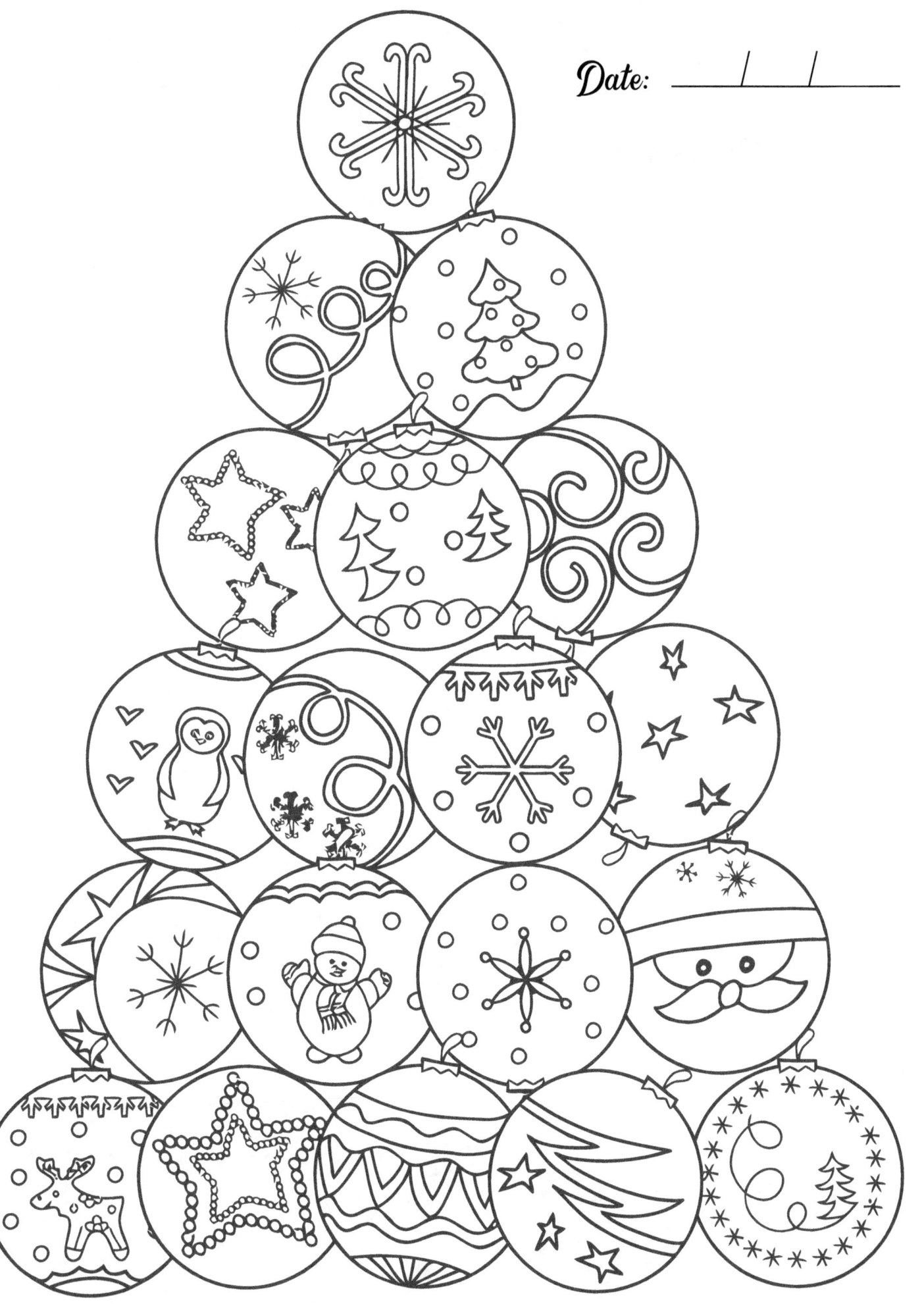

Date: _____ / _____ / _____

Write and Draw to Express Yourself

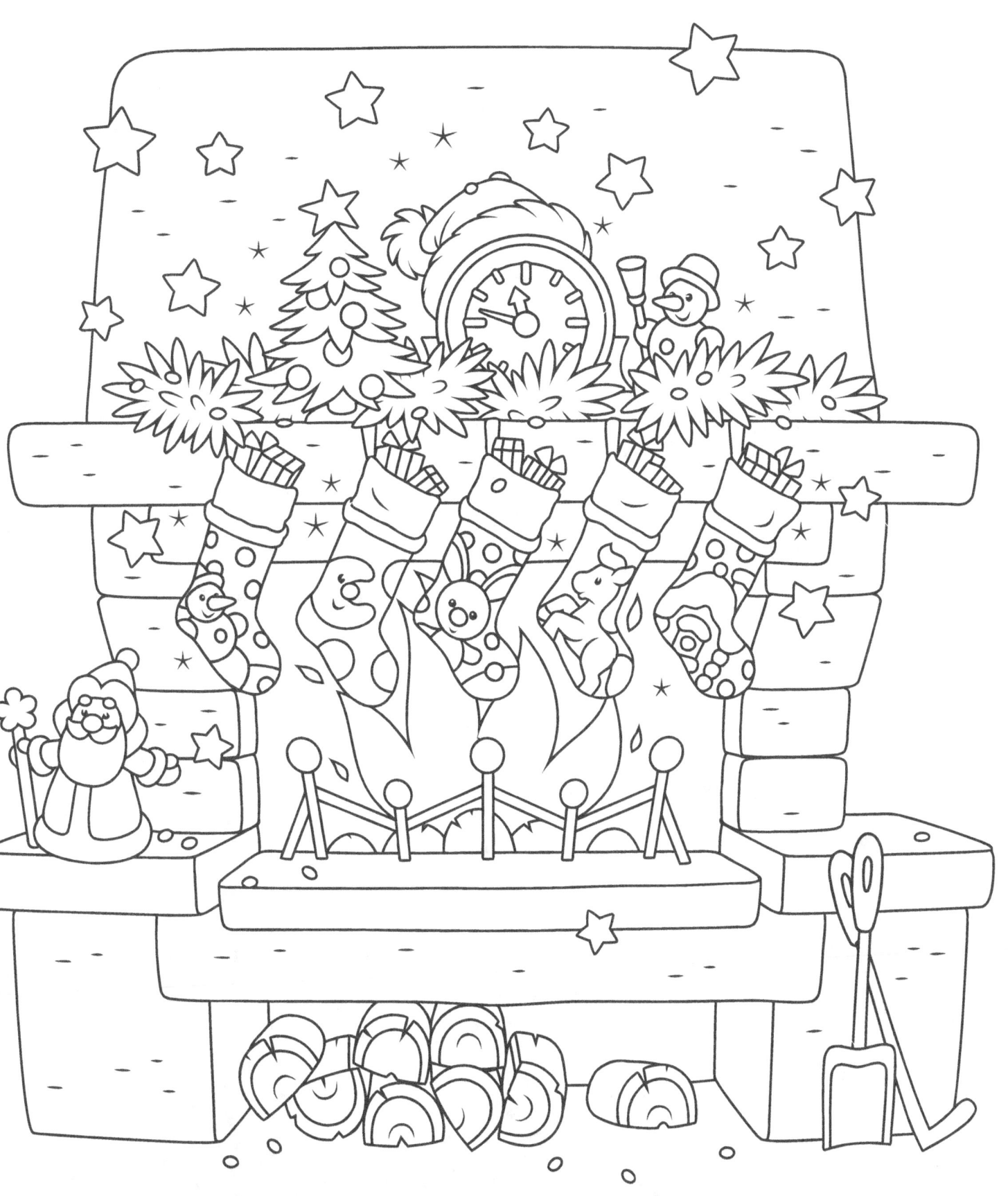

Write and Draw to Express Yourself

Date: _____/____/_____

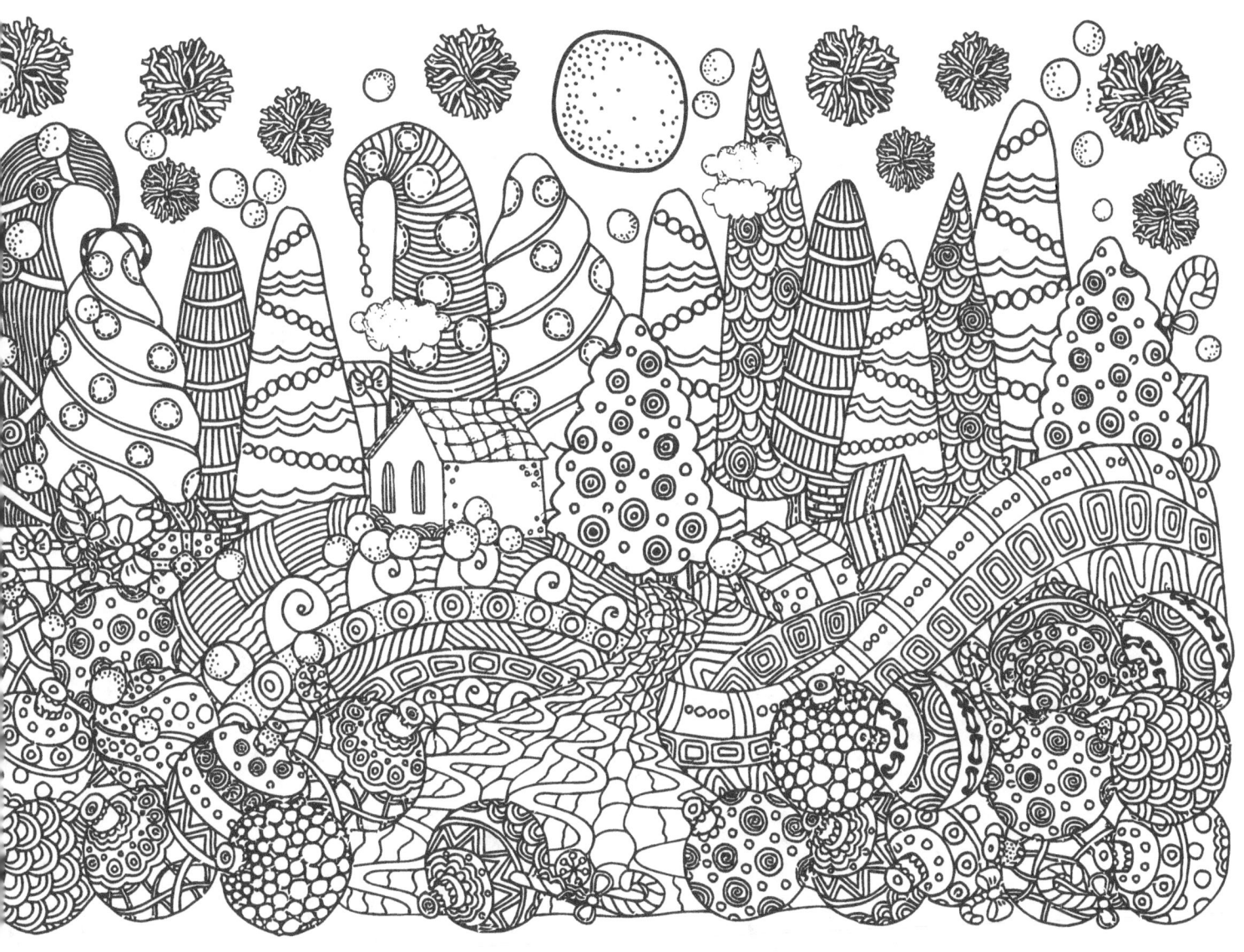

Write and Draw to Express Yourself

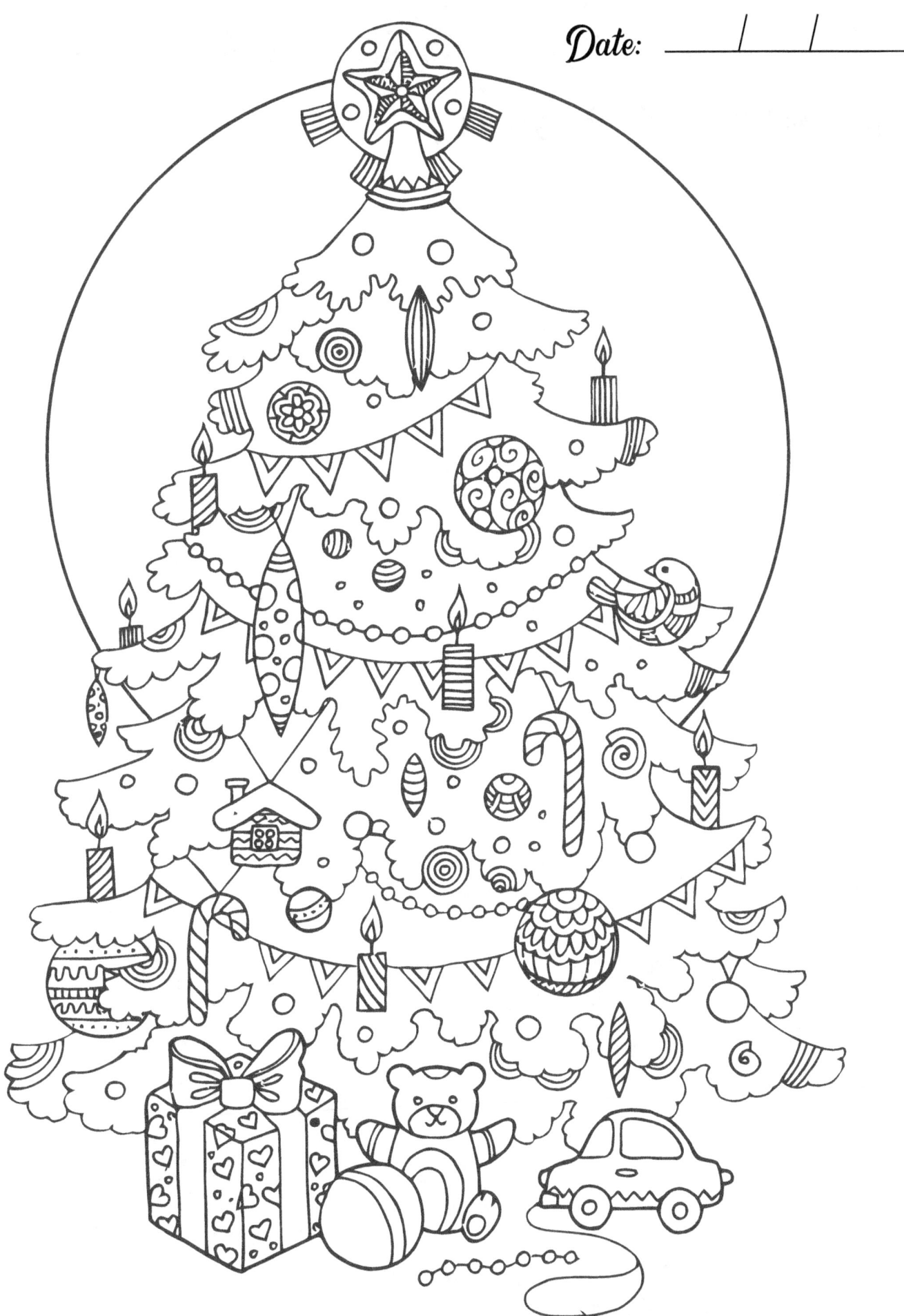

Write and Draw to Express Yourself

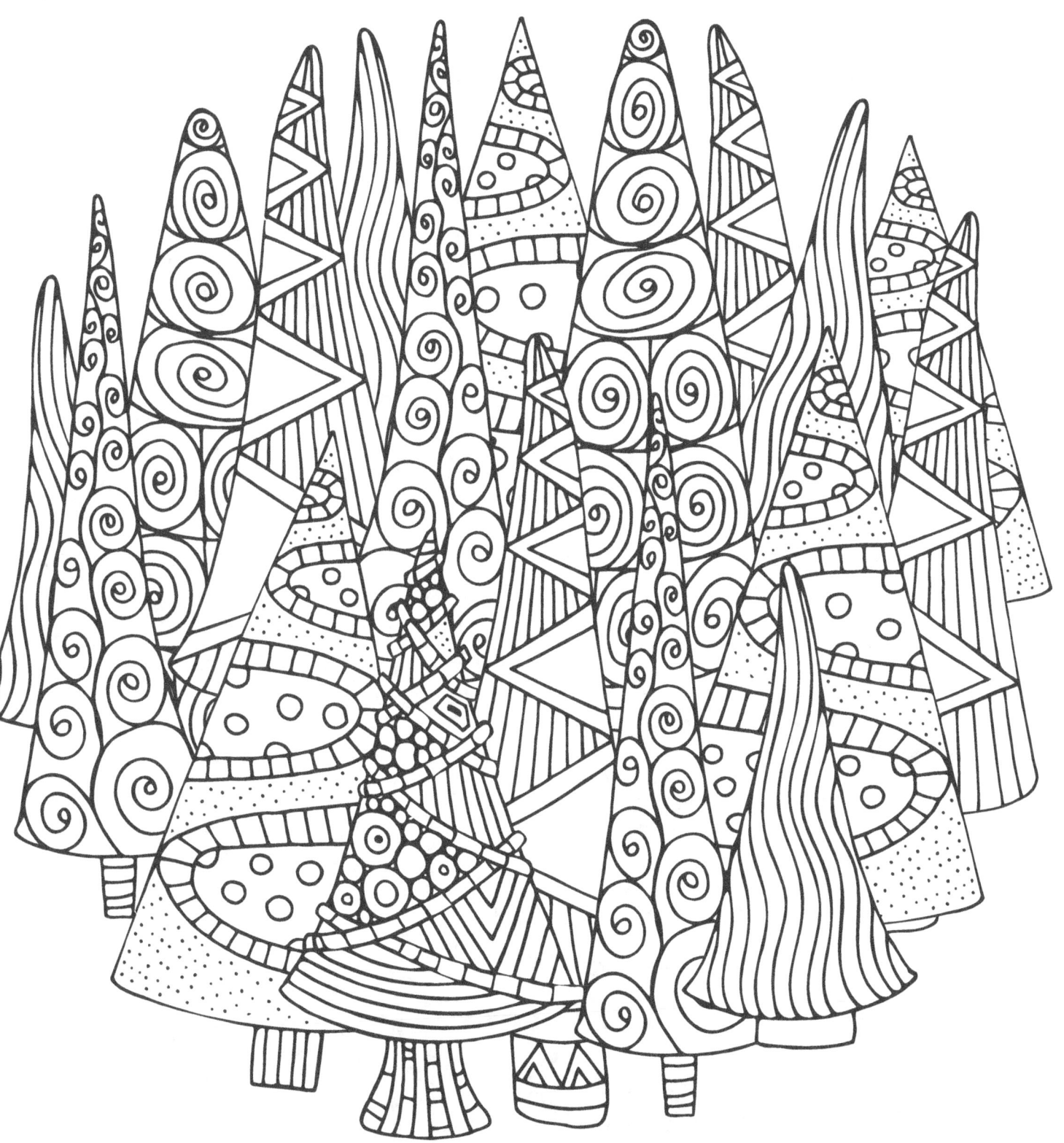

Write and Draw to Express Yourself

Date: ___/___/___

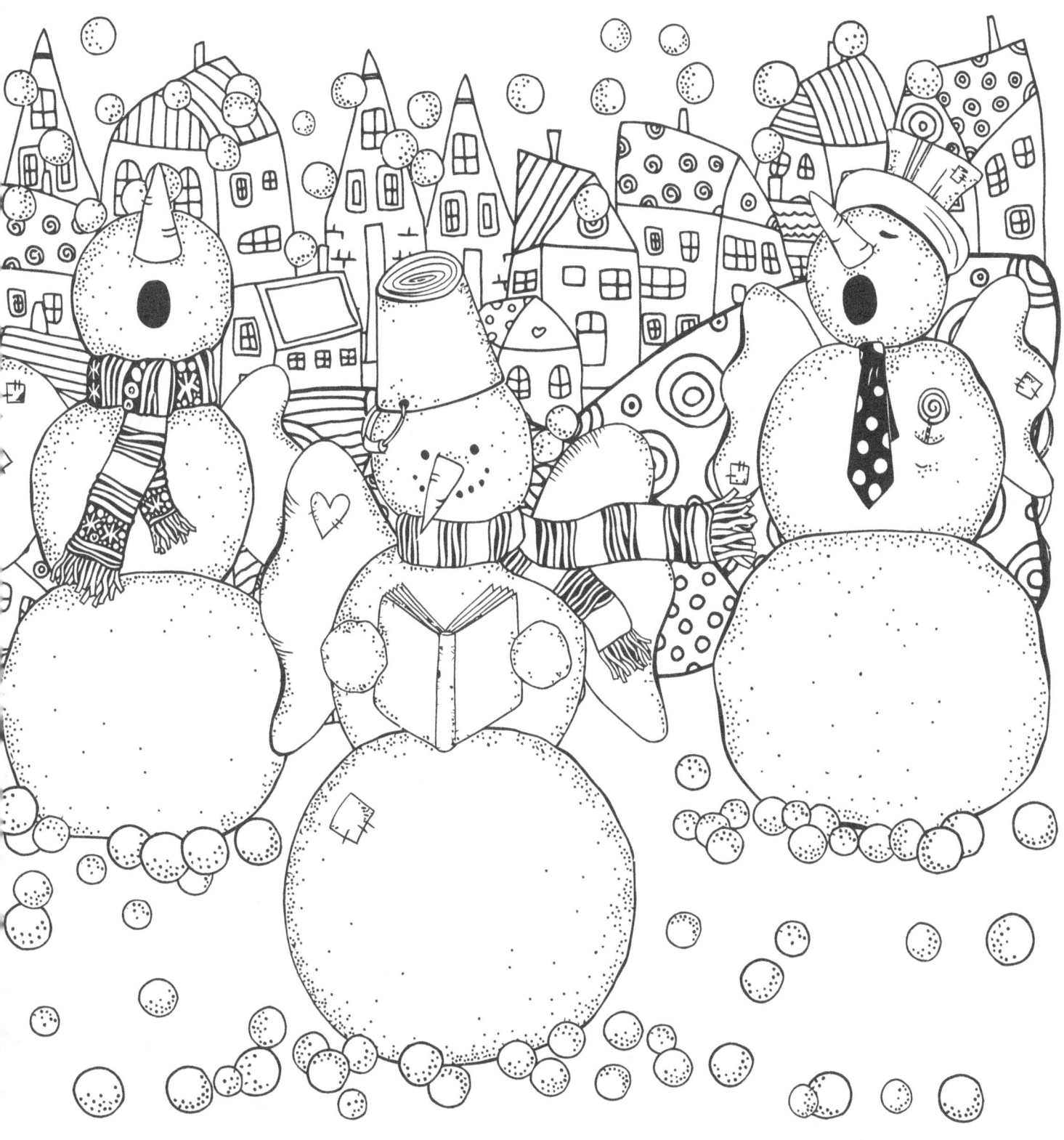

Write and Draw to Express Yourself

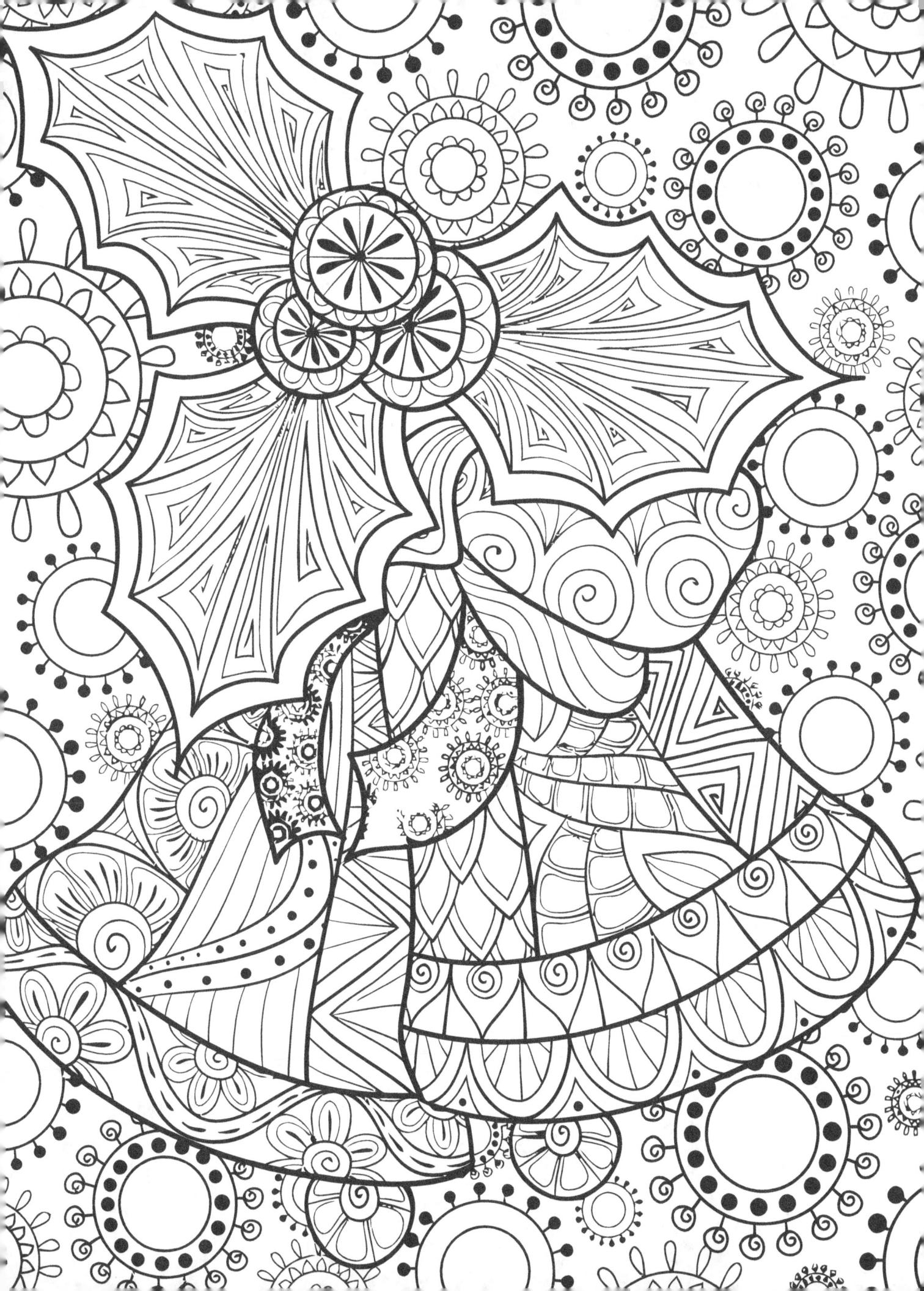

Write and Draw to Express Yourself

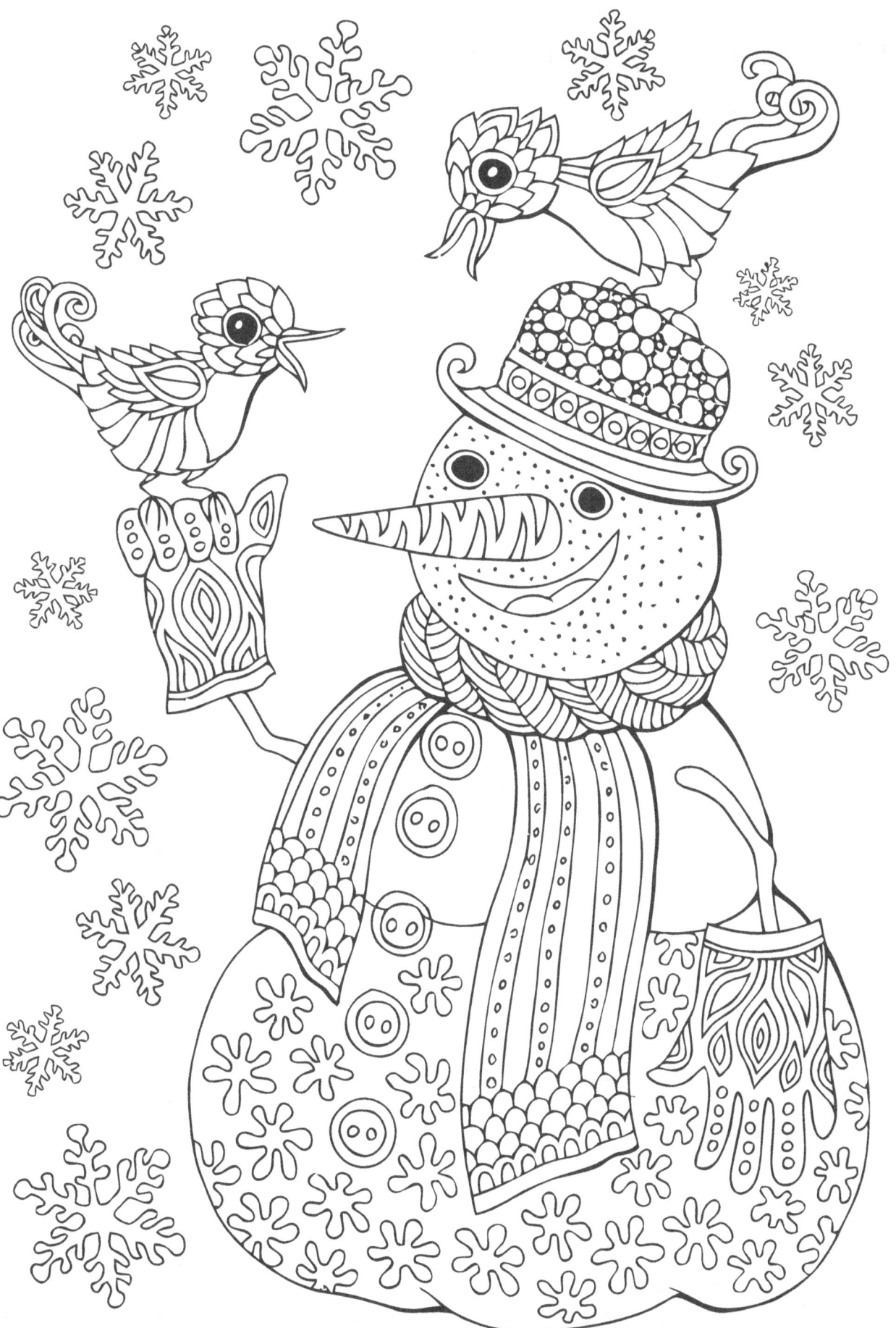

Write and Draw to Express Yourself

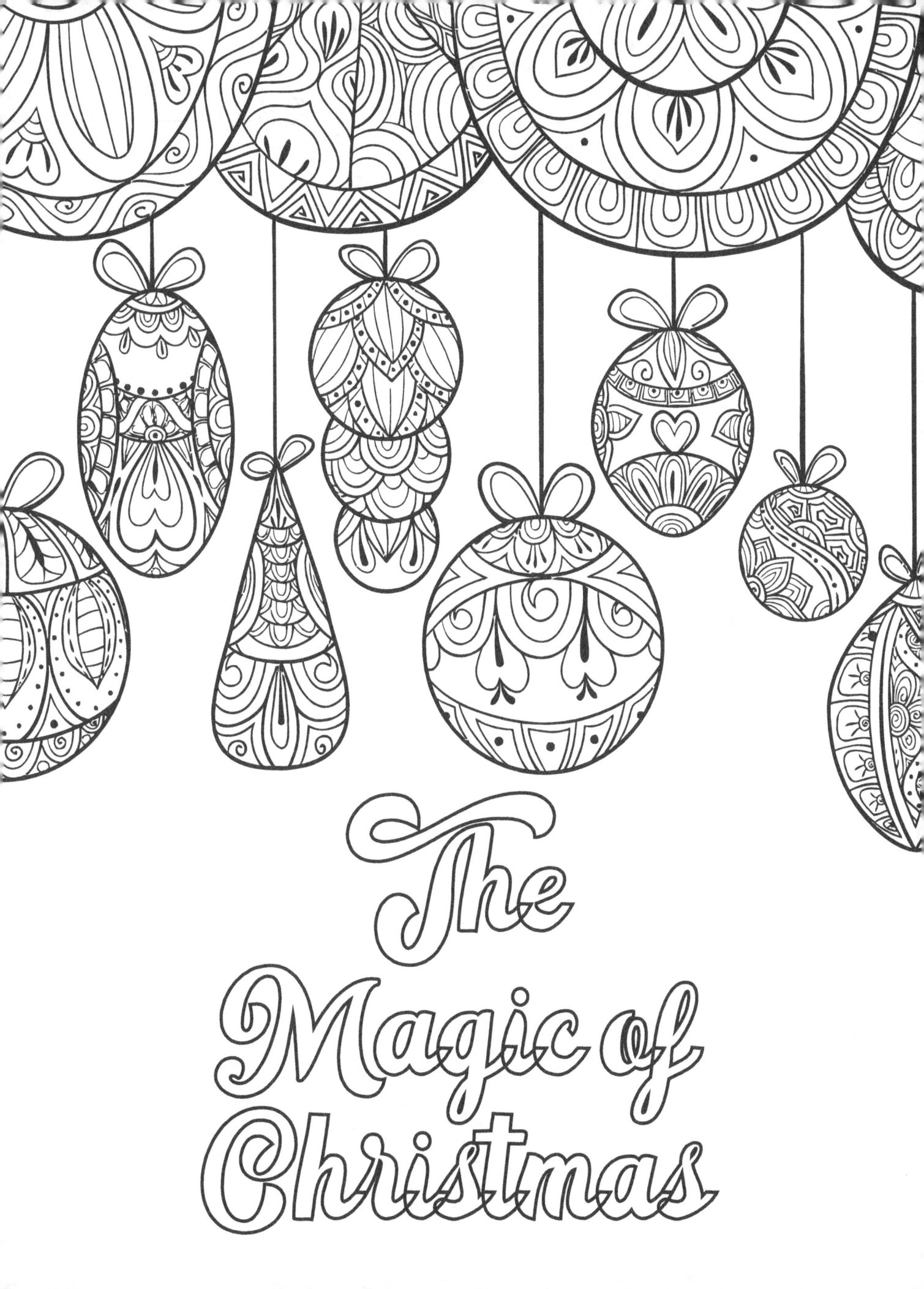

Write and Draw to Express Yourself

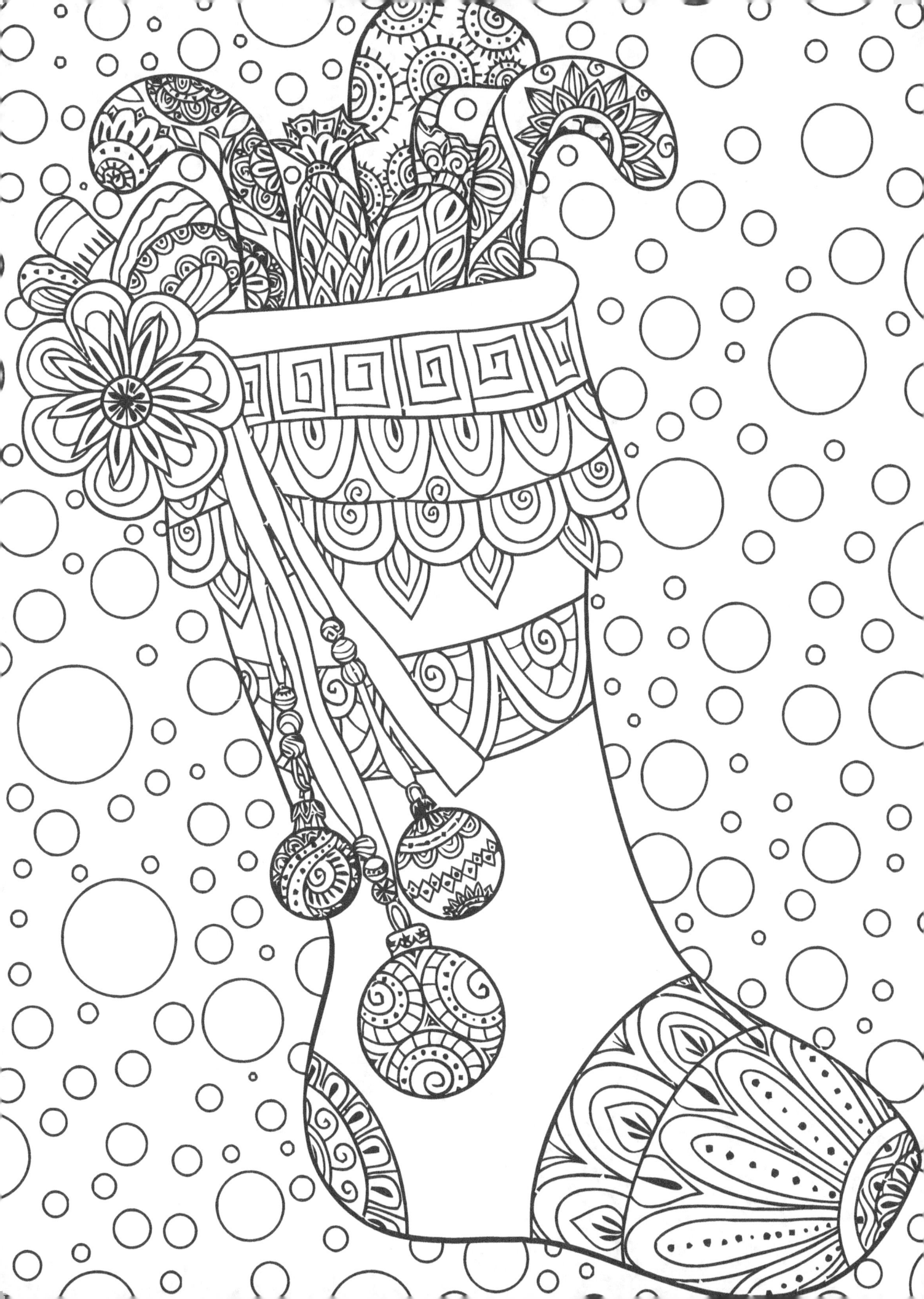

Write and Draw to Express Yourself

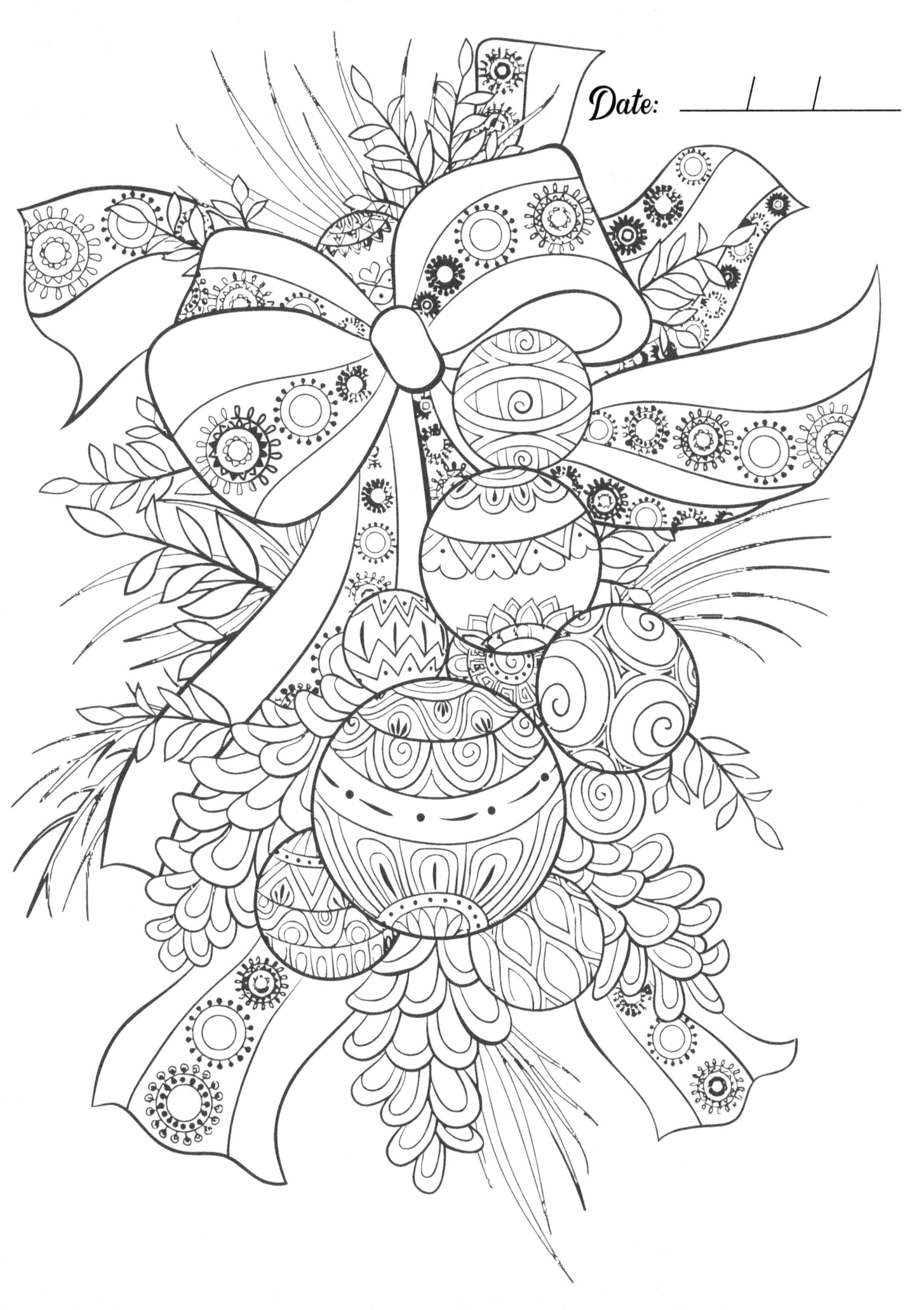

Date: _____ / _____ / _____

Write and Draw to Express Yourself

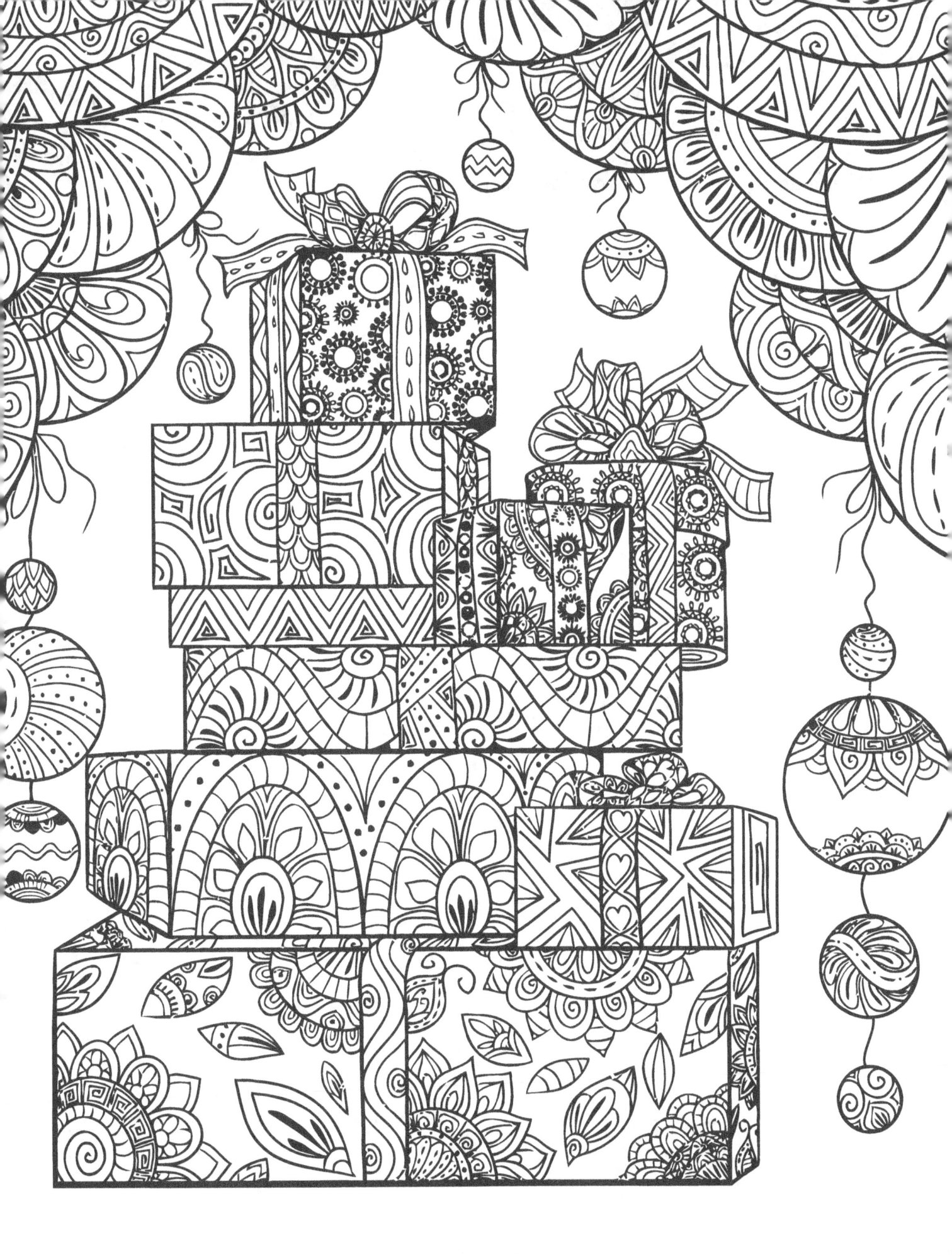

Write and Draw to Express Yourself

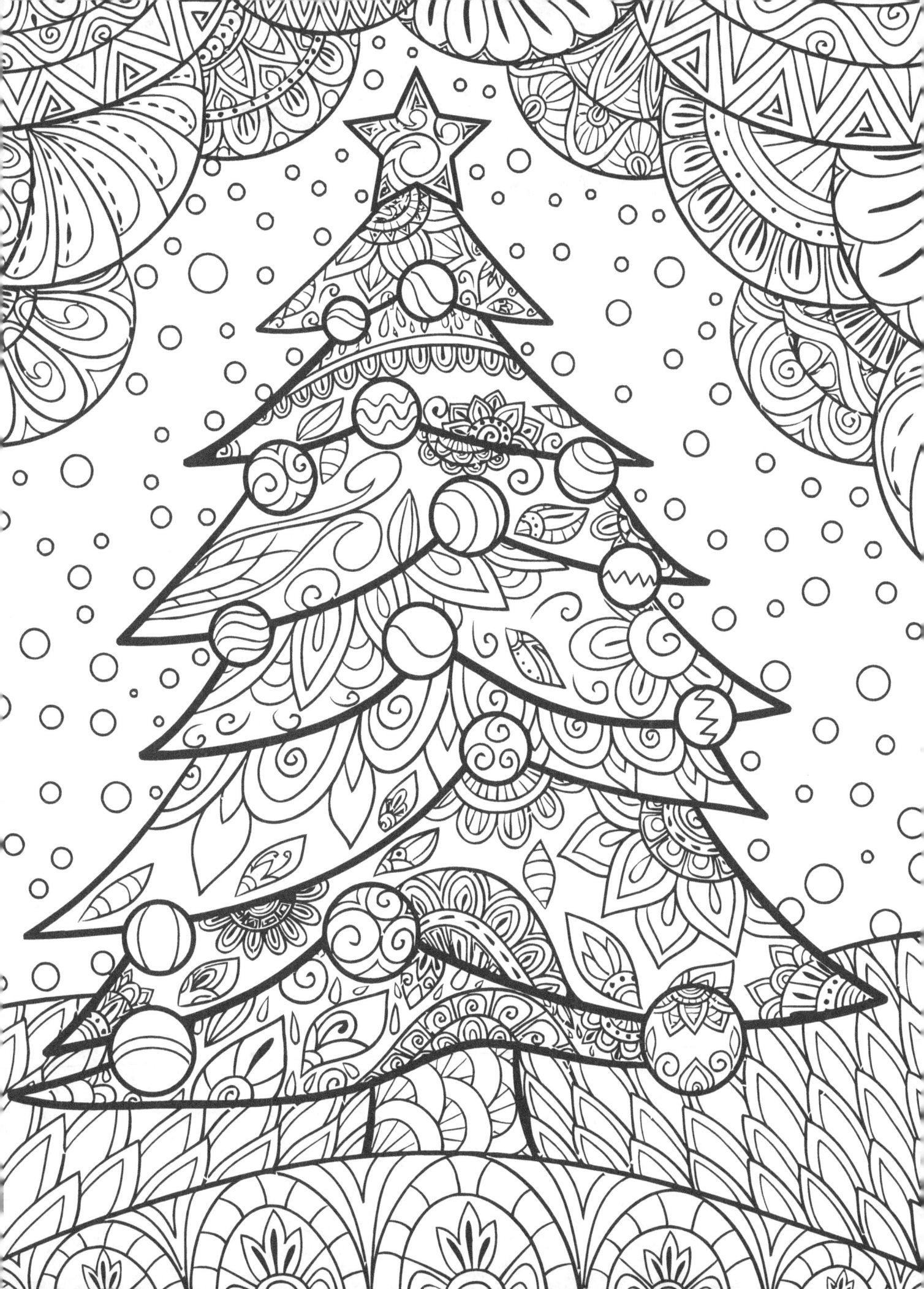

Date: ___/___/___

Write and Draw to Express Yourself

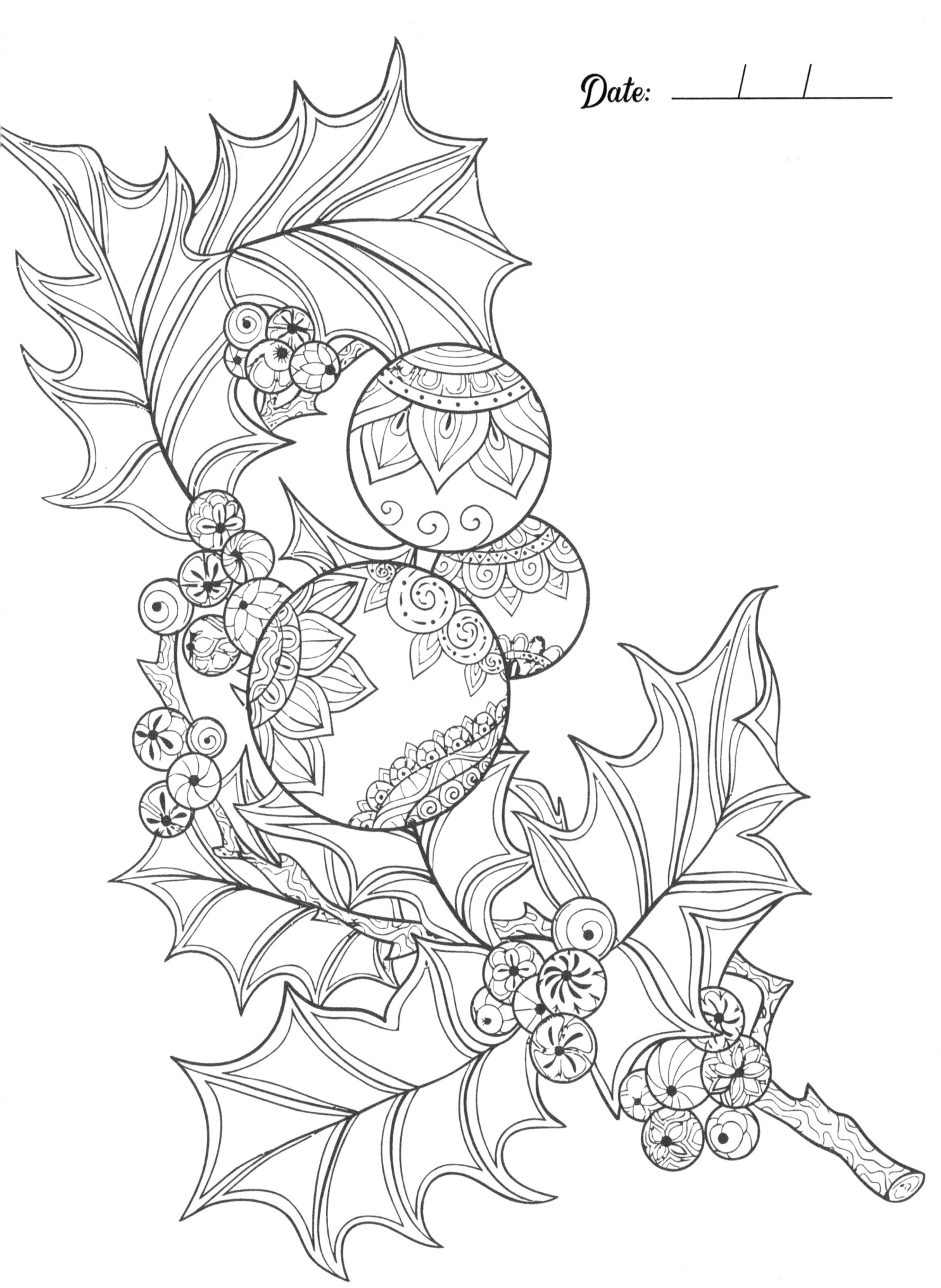

Write and Draw to Express Yourself

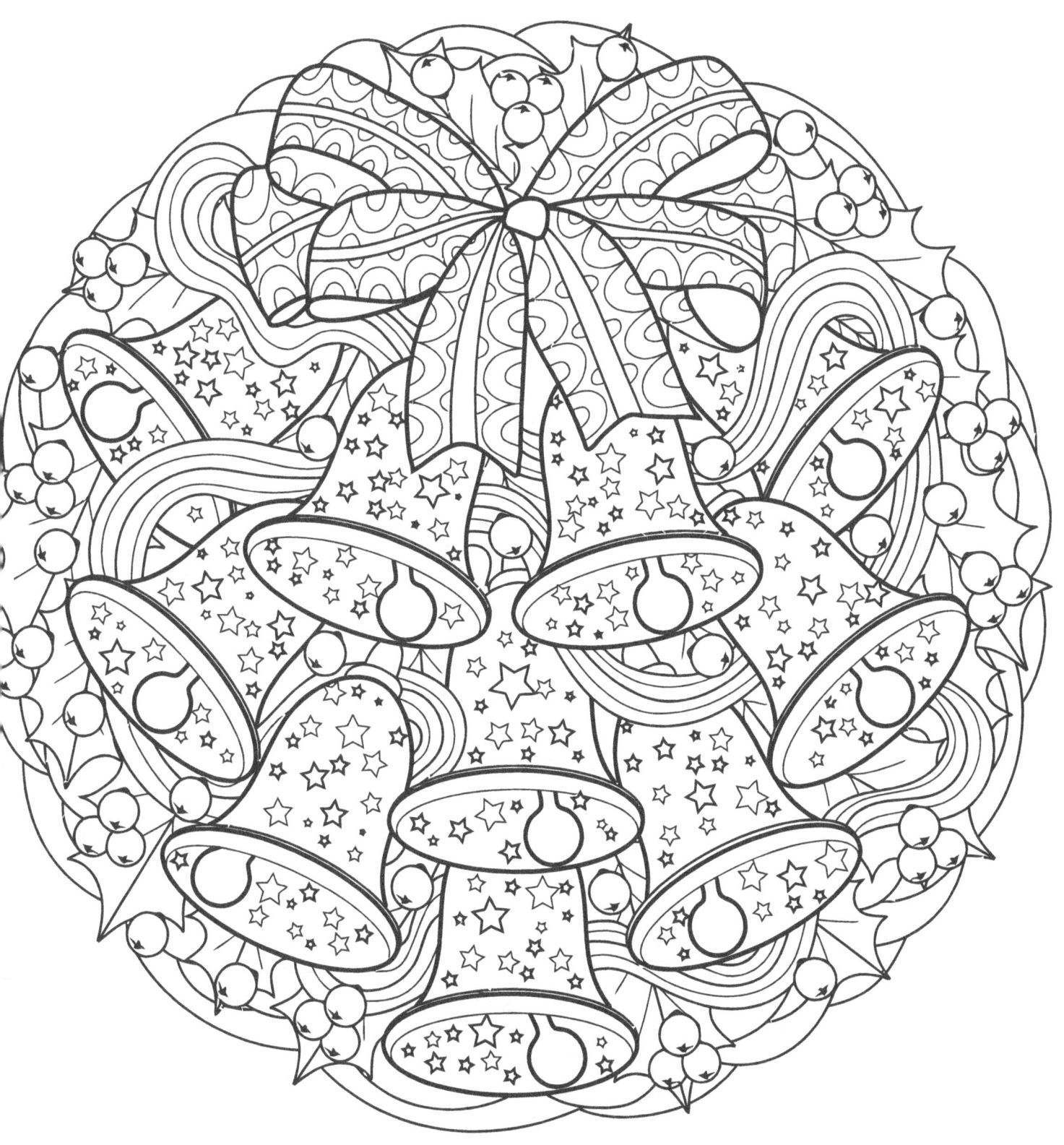

Write and Draw to Express Yourself

Write and Draw to Express Yourself

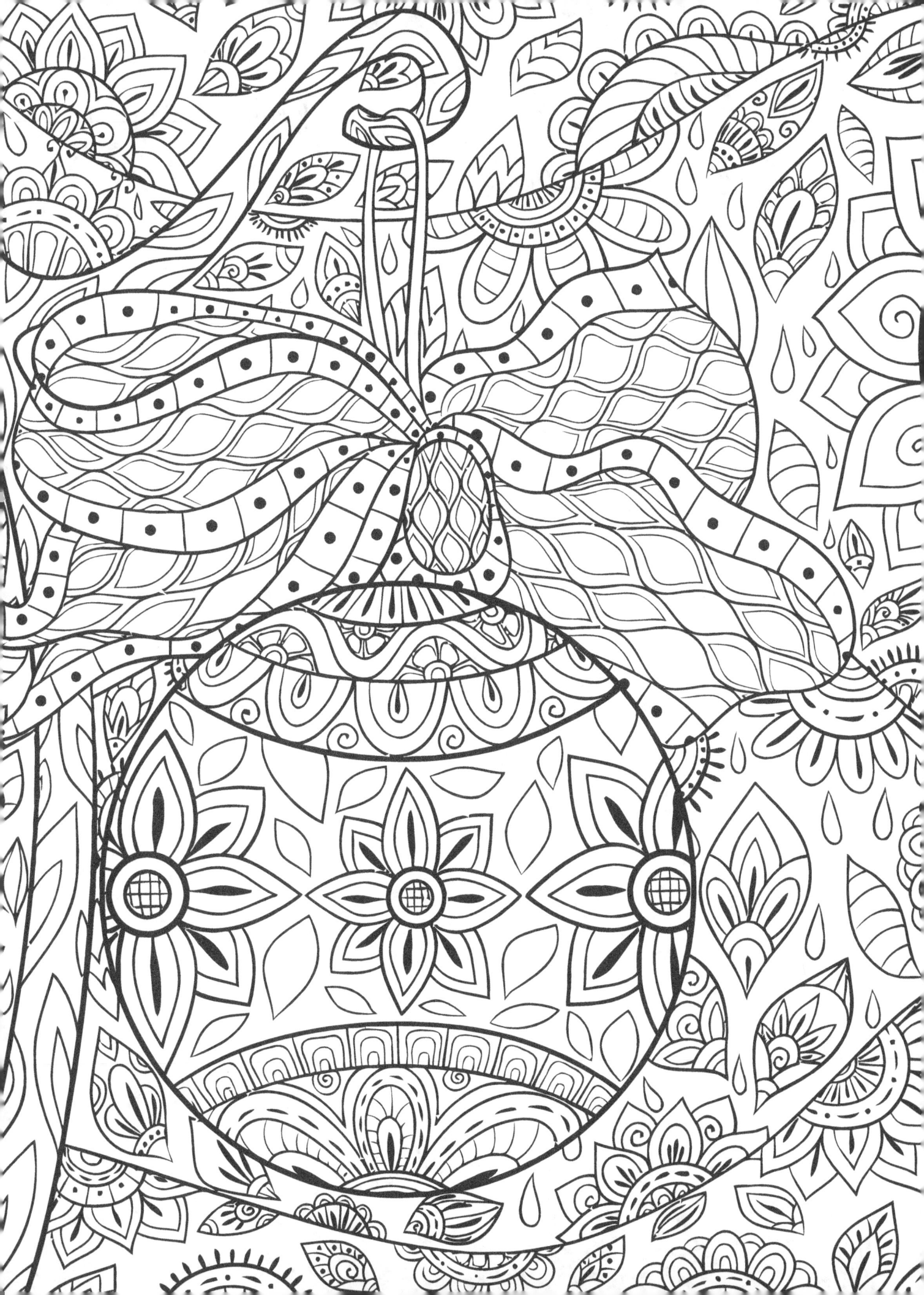

Write and Draw to Express Yourself

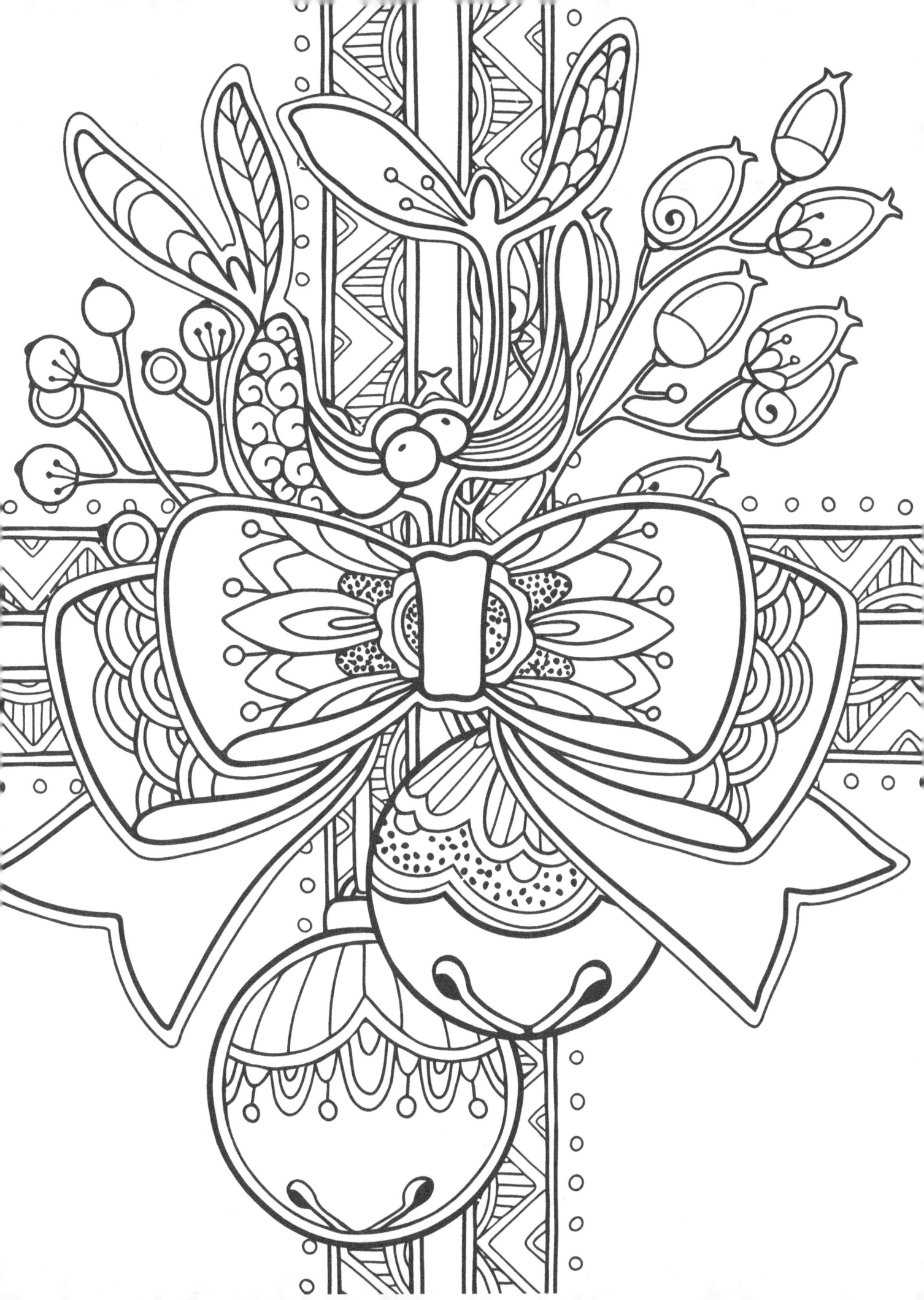

Write and Draw to Express Yourself

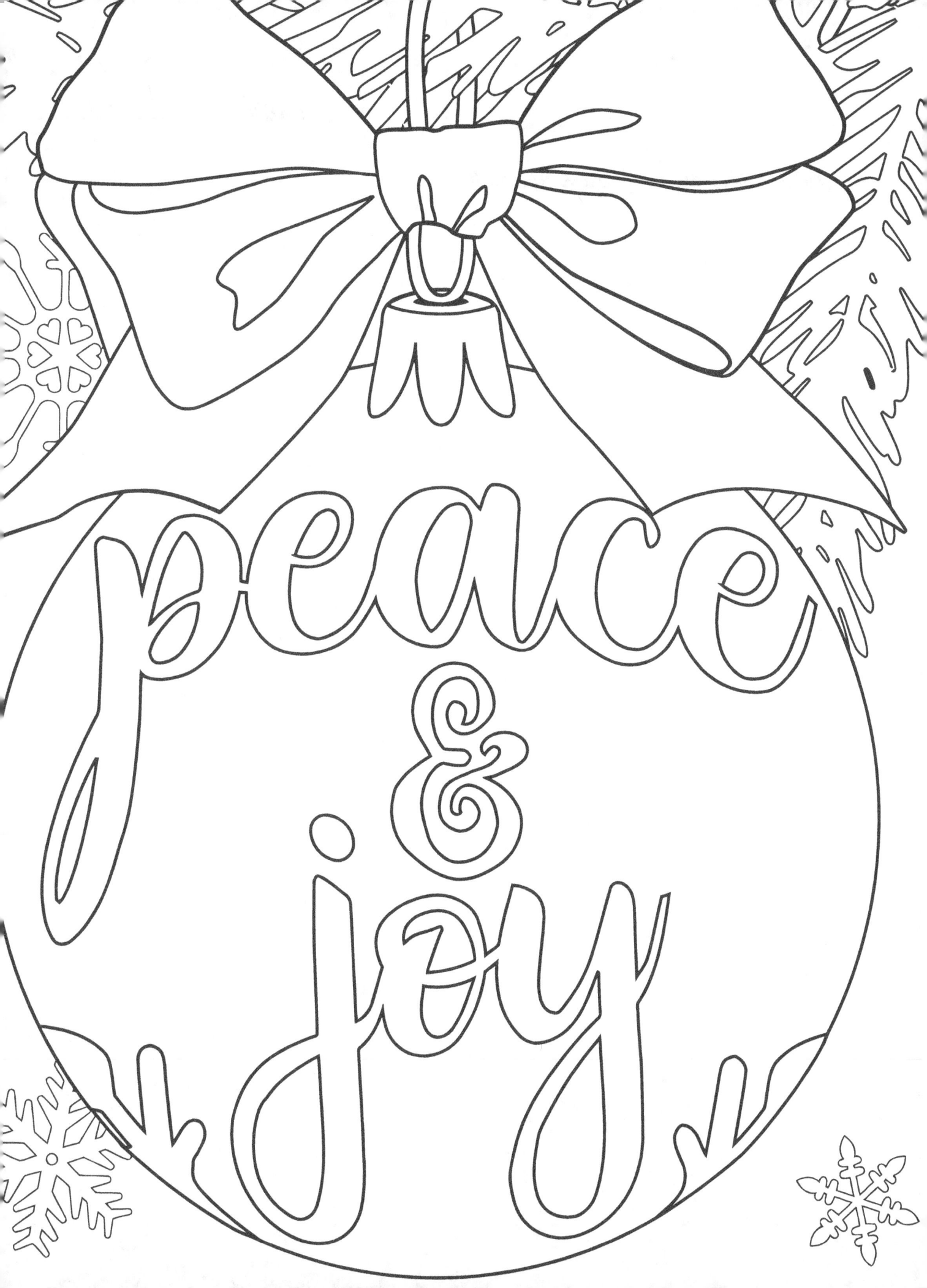

Write and Draw to Express Yourself

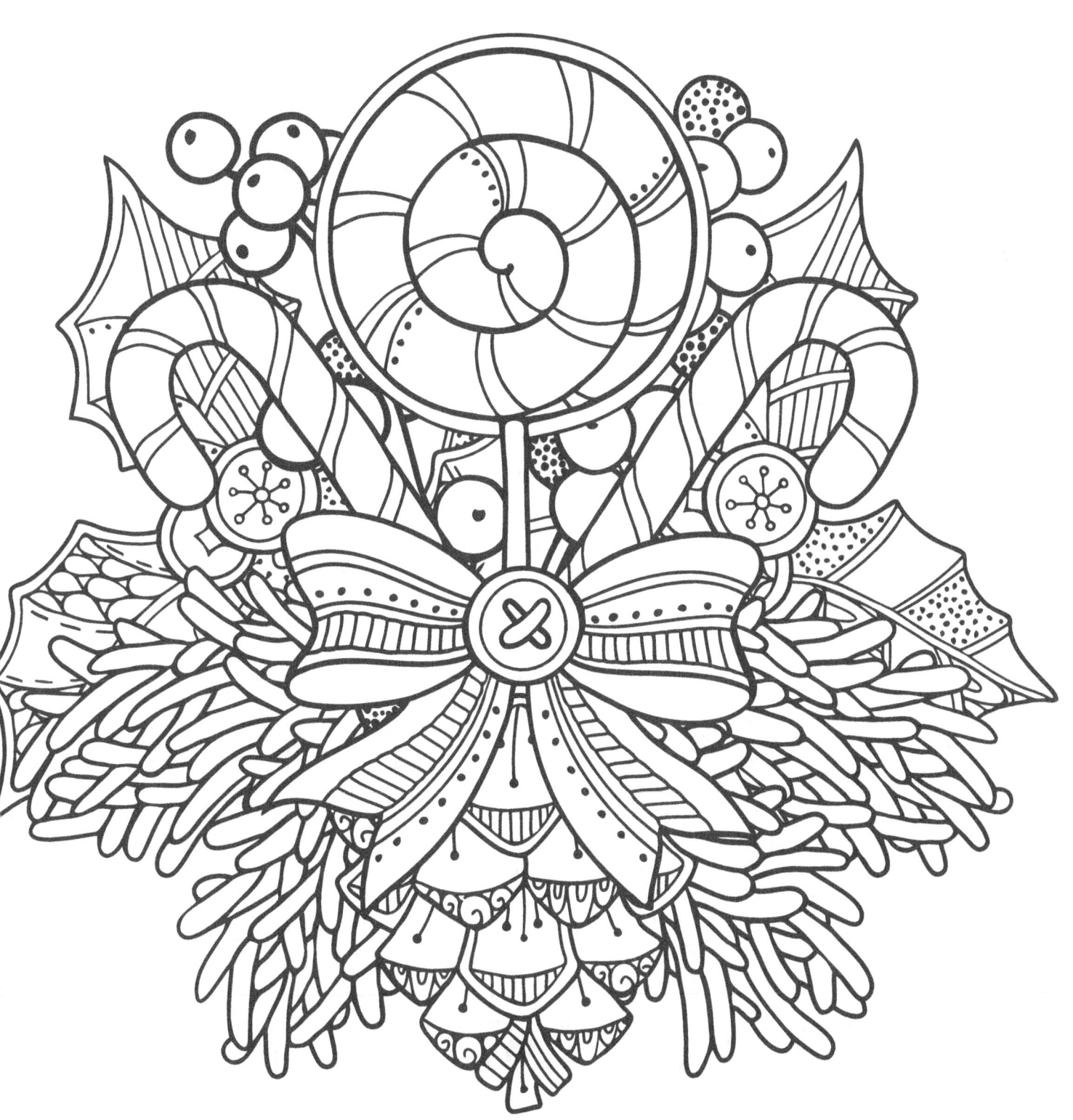

Write and Draw to Express Yourself

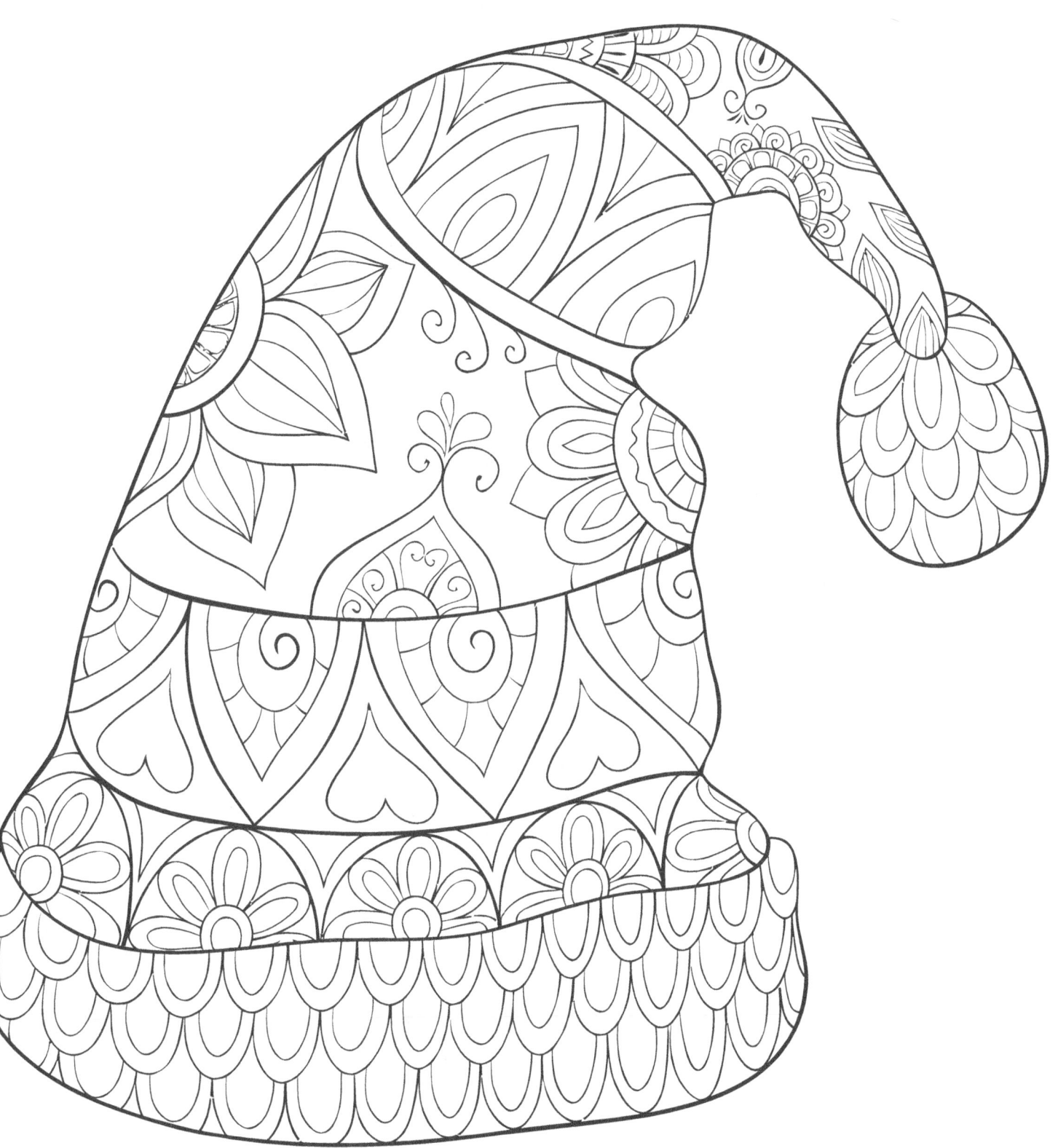

Write and Draw to Express Yourself

Date: _____ / _____ / _____

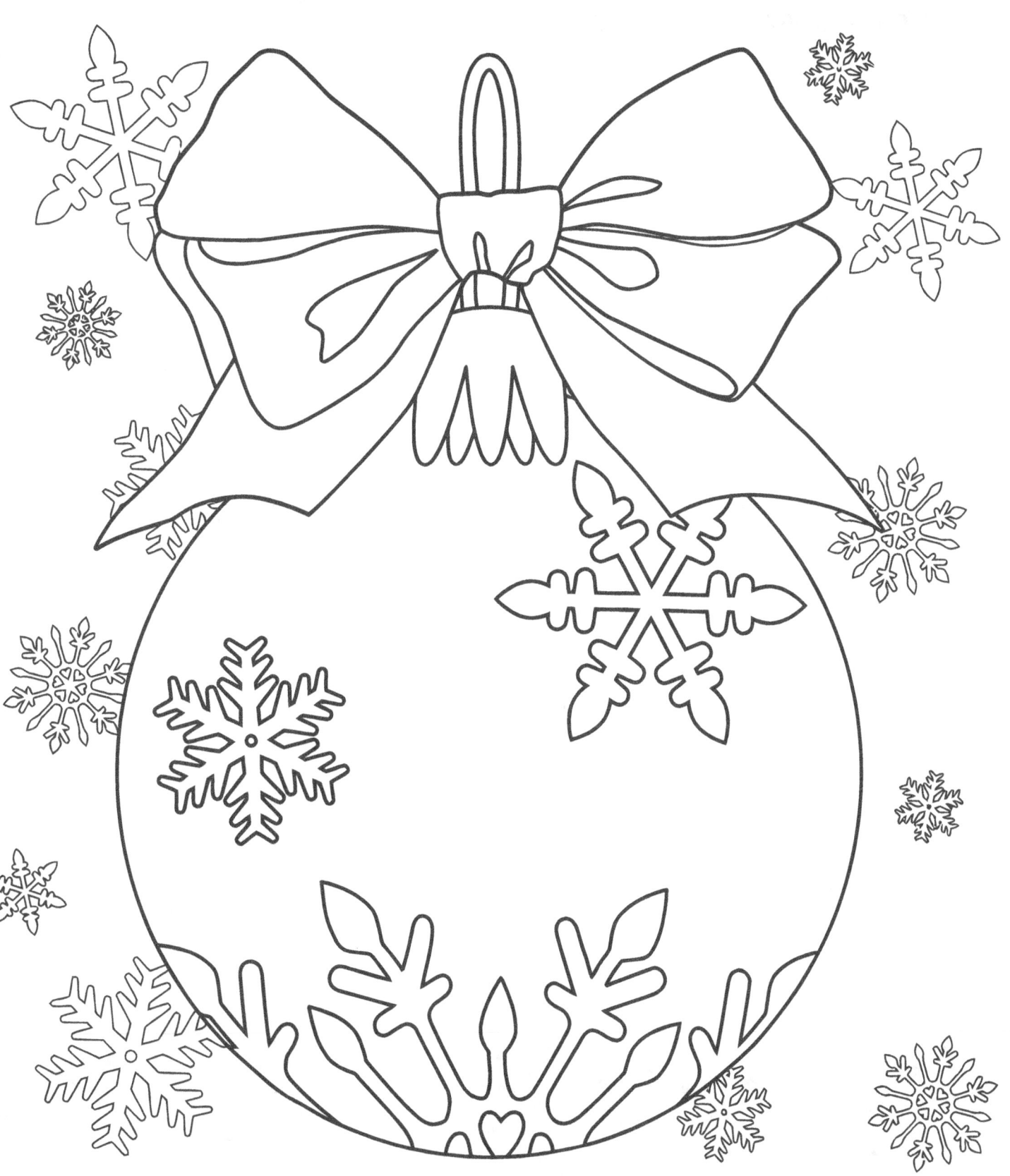

Write and Draw to Express Yourself

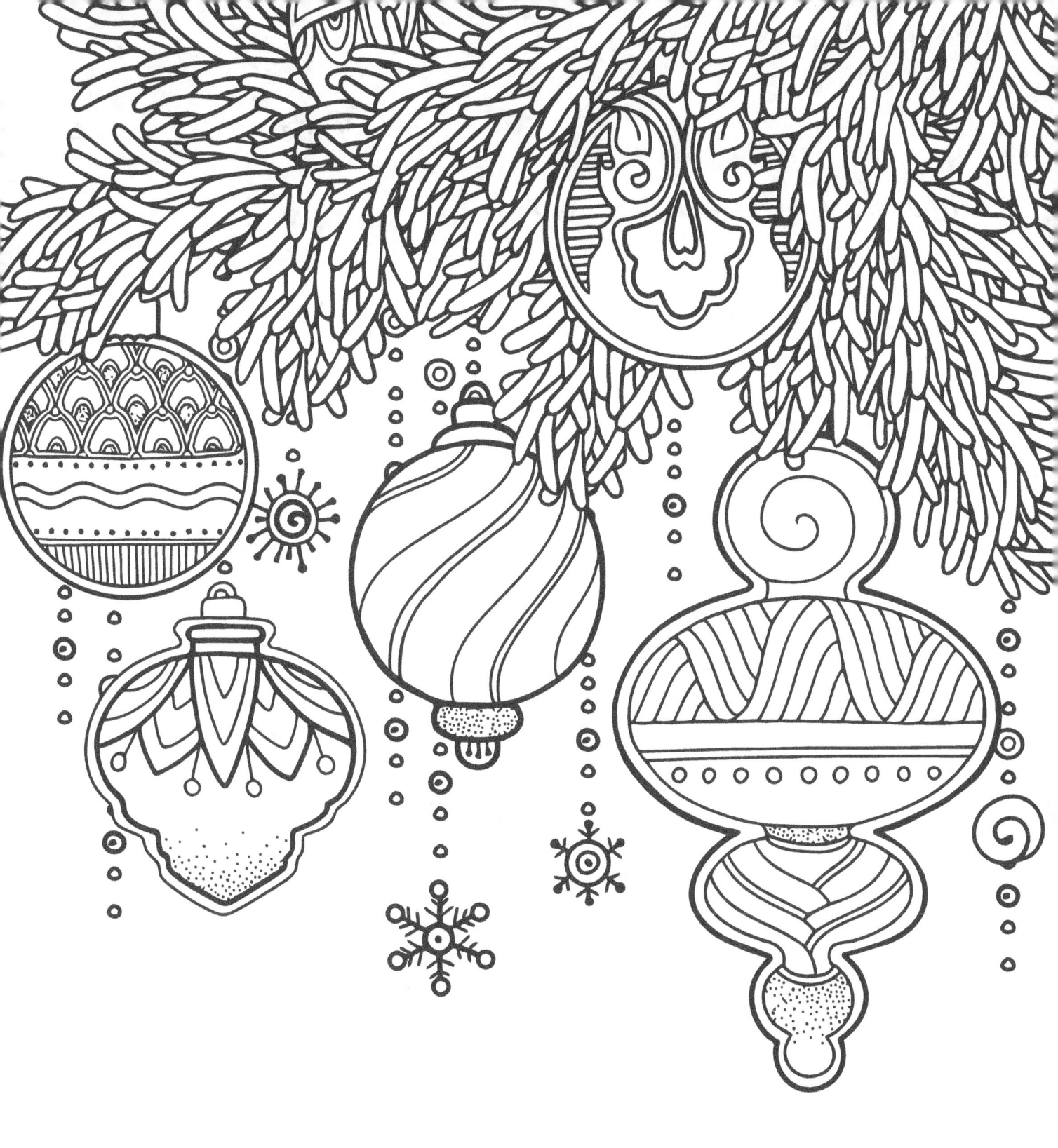

Write and Draw to Express Yourself

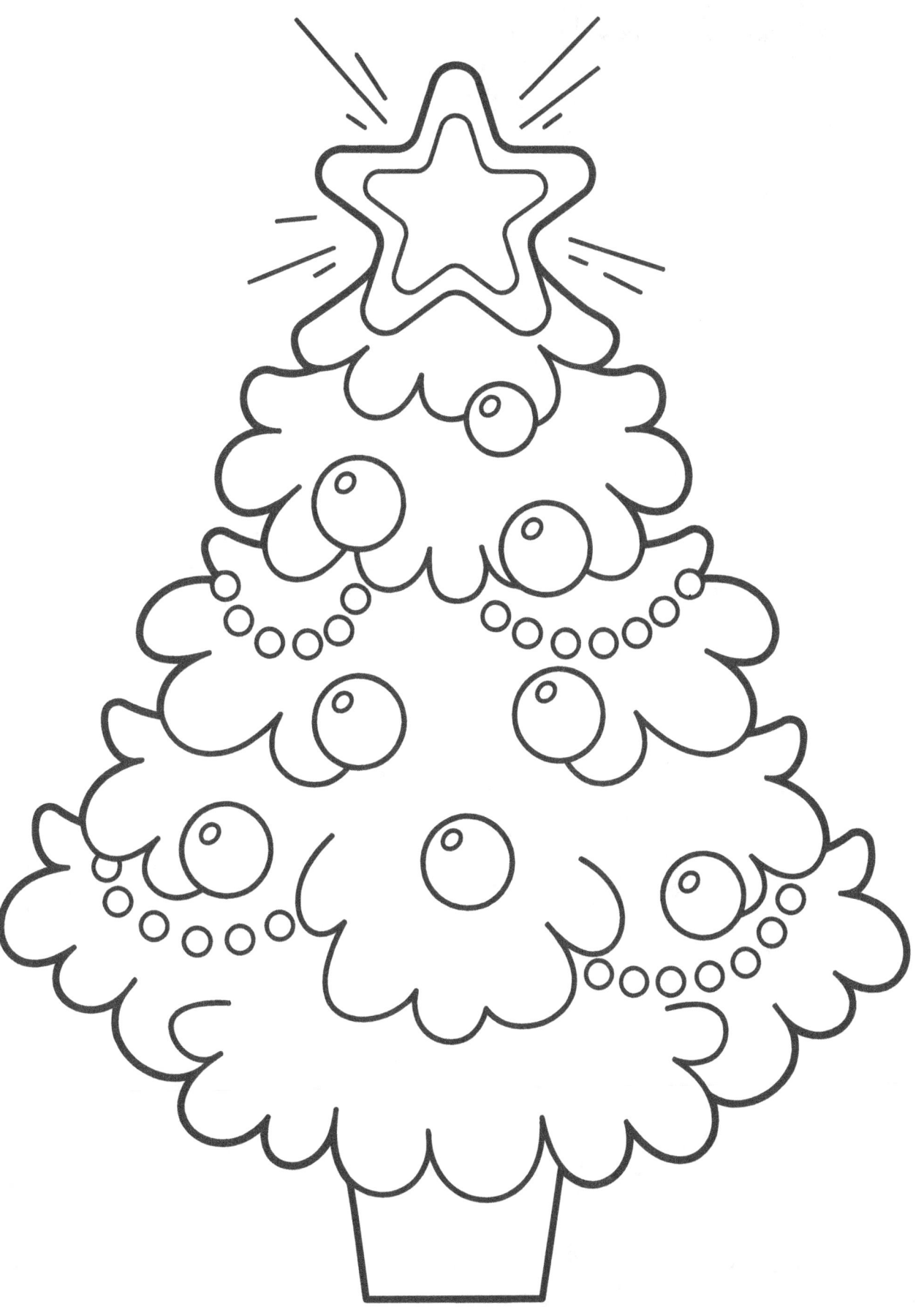

Write and Draw to Express Yourself

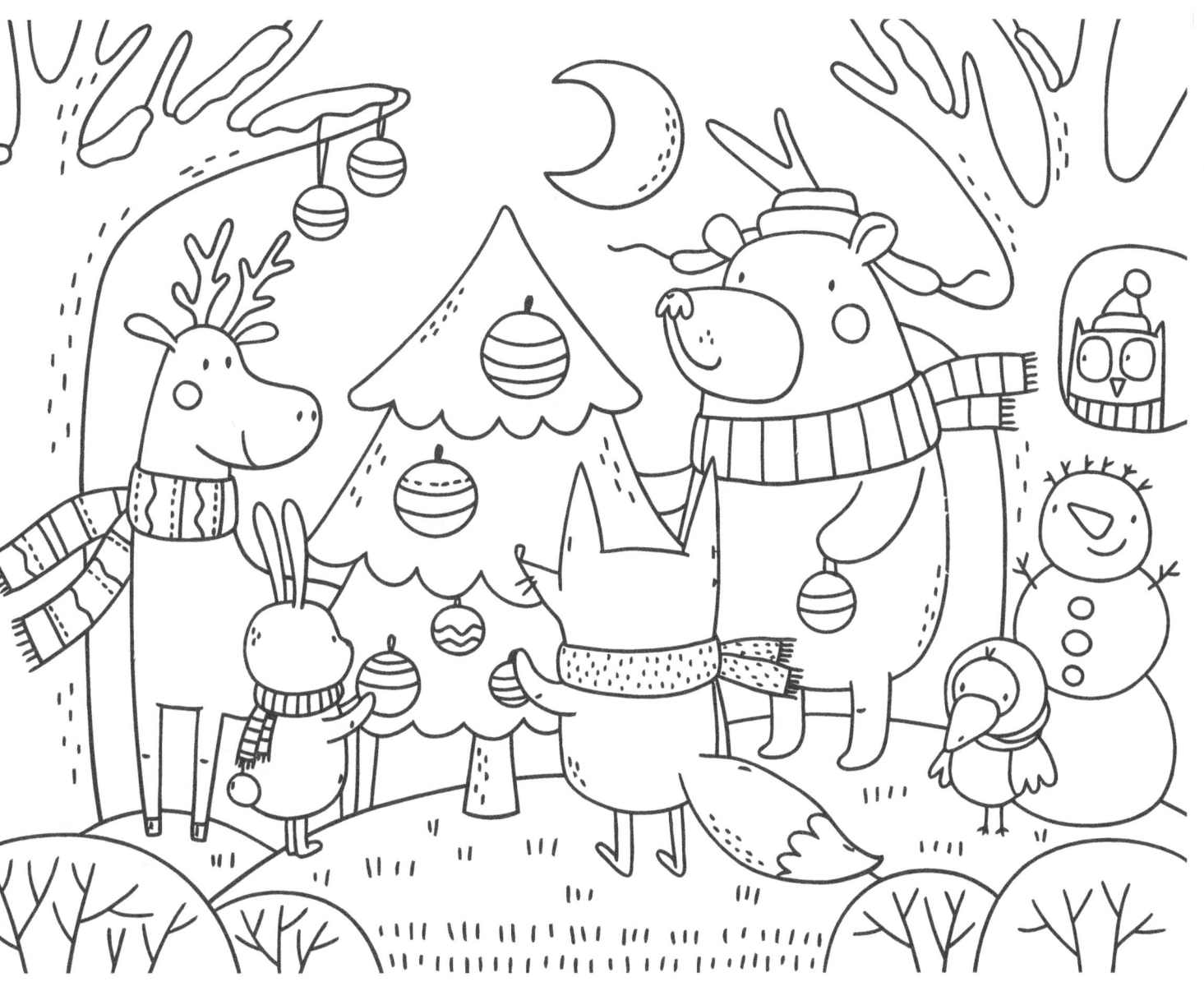

Write and Draw to Express Yourself

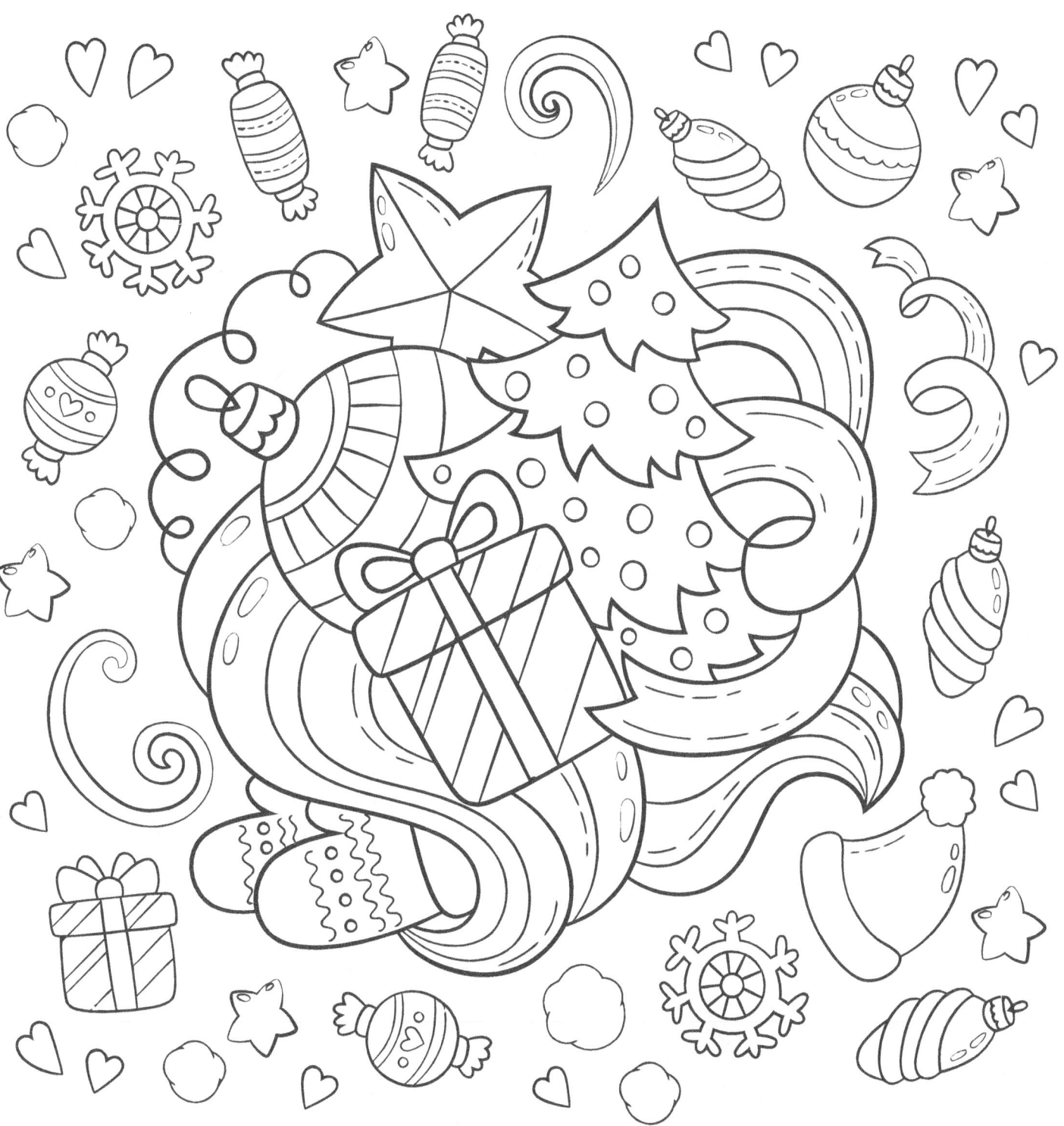

Write and Draw to Express Yourself

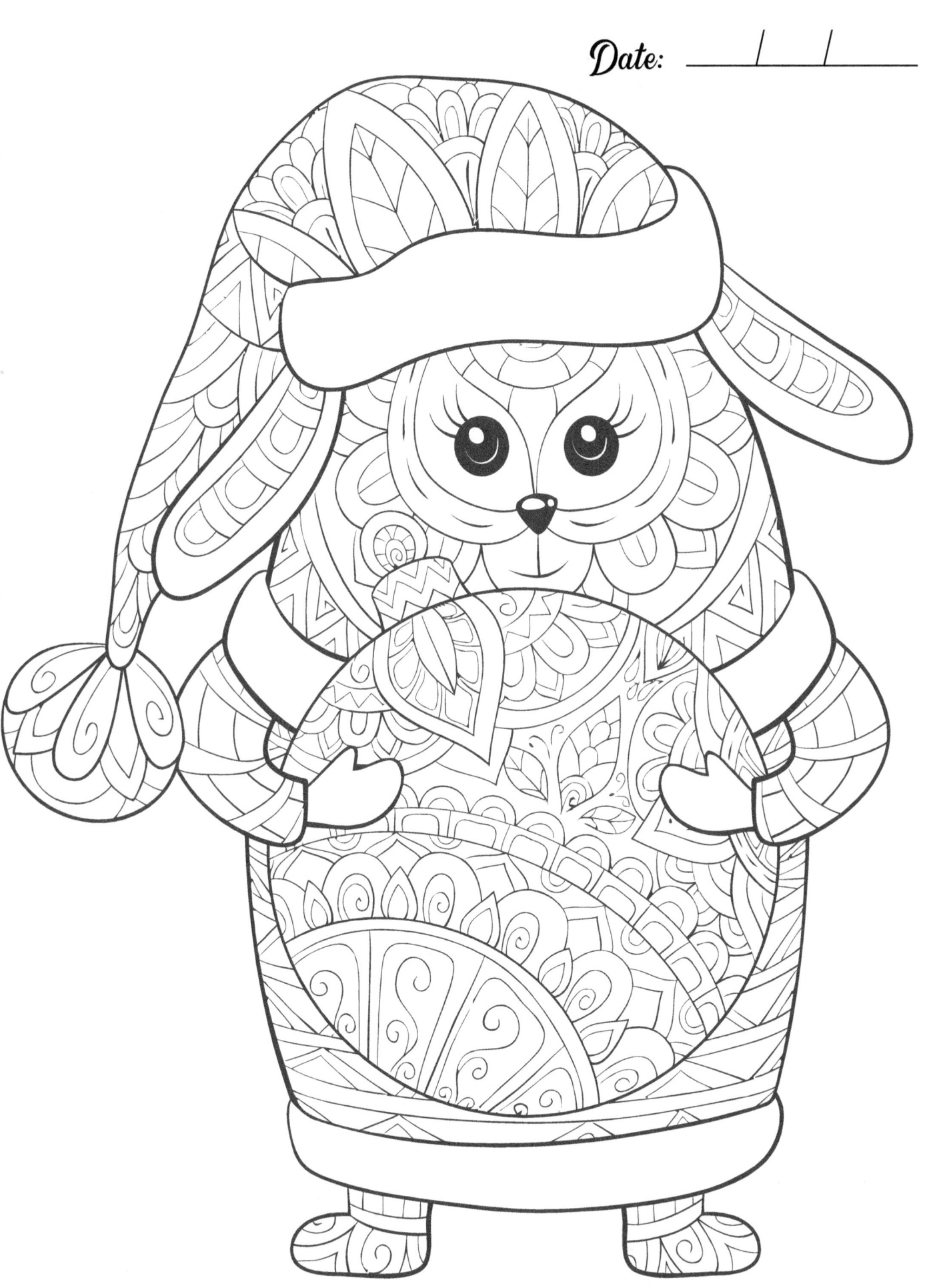